Logbook
Foundation Course

For First MBBS Students

Logbook Foundation Course

For First MBBS Students

Yogesh D MBBS MD (Anatomy)
Assistant Professor
Basaveshwara Medical College and Hospital
Chitradurga

JAYPEE

JAYPEE BROTHERS MEDICAL PUBLISHERS

The Health Sciences Publisher

New Delhi | London

JAYPEE **Jaypee Brothers Medical Publishers (P) Ltd**

Headquarters
Jaypee Brothers Medical Publishers (P) Ltd
23/23-B, Ansari Road, Daryaganj
New Delhi 110 002, India
Phone:+91-11-23272143, +91-11-23272703
+91-11-23282021, +91-11-23245672
E-mail: jaypee@jaypeebrothers.com

Corporate Office
Jaypee Brothers Medical Publishers (P) Ltd.
4838/24, Ansari Road, Daryaganj
New Delhi 110 002, India
Phone: +91-11-43574357
Fax: +91-11-43574314
E-mail: jaypee@jaypeebrothers.com

Overseas Office
JP Medical Ltd
83 Victoria Street, London
SW1H 0HW (UK)
Phone: +44 20 3170 8910
E-mail: info@jpmedpub.com

EU GPSR Authorised Representative
Logos Europe, 9 rue Nicolas Poussin
17000, La Rochelle, France
Phone: +33 (0) 6 67 93 73 78
E-mail: Contact@logoseurope.eu

Website: www.jaypeebrothers.com
Website: www.jaypeedigital.com

Inquiries for bulk sales may be solicited at: jaypee@jaypeebrothers.com

Logbook–Foundation Course (For First MBBS Students)

First Edition: ***2020***

Reprint: 2024, **2025**

ISBN: 978-93-89188-82-0

Printed at: Sterling Graphics Pvt. Ltd.

THIS IS TO CERTIFY THAT THIS IS A BONA FIDE WORK DONE BY ____________ AS PART OF THE FOUNDATION COURSE FOR FIRST YEAR MBBS DURING THE

YEAR 20_____ TO 20_____.

HIS/HER WORK IS COMPLETE, AND THE STUDENT HAS ATTAINED THE REQUISITE COMPETENCIES AS PRESCRIBED UNDER THE FOUNDATION COURSE.

Submitted for University Examination in the year of ____________________

________________________	____________________________
Signature of the Teacher in-charge	Signature of the Foundation Course in-Charge
________________________	_____________________
Signature of the Examiner	Signature of the Examiner

Preface

This logbook is intended for the use of first year medical students who join MBBS course from the year 2019 and is prepared as per the guidelines for implementation of foundation course as per Graduate Medical Education Regulations.

This logbook will help you record your opinions on the topics covered, the teaching methods used and reflect on the specific topics that you have learnt in a specific session and will enable your teachers to better evaluate the teaching methods to help you achieve your competencies and learning outcomes.

Date: 02/08/2019

Dr Yogesh D MBBS, MD(Anatomy)
Assistant Professor of Anatomy
Basaveshwara Medical College and Hospital
Chitradurga

Contents

Foundation Course Modules

1. **Orientation Module** **Total hours: 30**
   - **1A.** Orientation Module: Introduction to institution / campus / facilities
   - **1B.** Orientation Module: Role of doctors in the society
   - **1C.** Orientation Module: History of Medicine and alternate systems
   - **1D.** Orientation Module: IMG roles / overview MBBS curriculum various career pathways
   - **1E.** Orientation Module: Principles of family practice
2. **Skills Module:** **Total hours: 35**
   - **2A.** Skills Module: First Aid
   - **2B.** Skills Module: BLS
   - **2C.** Skills Module: Universal precautions
   - **2D.** Skills Module: Waste management
   - **2E.** Skills Module: Immunization
   - **2F.** Skills Module: Documentation
3. **Community orientation module** **Total hours: 8**
   - **3A.** Community Orientation Module: National Health goals and policies/ health Care systems/community health
   - **3B.** Community Orientation Module: Interactions with patients and families, Communities.
4. **Professional Development and Ethics Module (P&E)** **Total hours: 40**
   - **4A.** (P&E): Concept of Professionalism and Ethics
   - **4B.** (P&E): White coat Ceremony
   - **4C.** (P&E): Professional behaviour and altruistic behaviour
   - **4D.** (P&E): Working in a health care team
   - **4E.** (P&E): Disability competencies
   - **4F.** (P&E): Cultural competence
   - **4G.** (P&E): Stress management
   - **4H.** (P&E): Time management
   - **4I.** (P&E): Interpersonal relationship
   - **4J.** (P&E): Learning
5. **Enhancement of Language and Computer Skills Module** **Total hours:40**
   - **5A.** Enhancement of Language and Computer Skills Module: Communication
   - **5B.** Enhancement of Language and Computer Skills Module: Local Language training
   - **5C.** Enhancement of Language and Computer Skills Module: English Language training
   - **5D.** Enhancement of Language and Computer Skills Module: Computer Skills training
6. **Sports and extracurricular activities:** **Total hours: 22**

Orientation Module

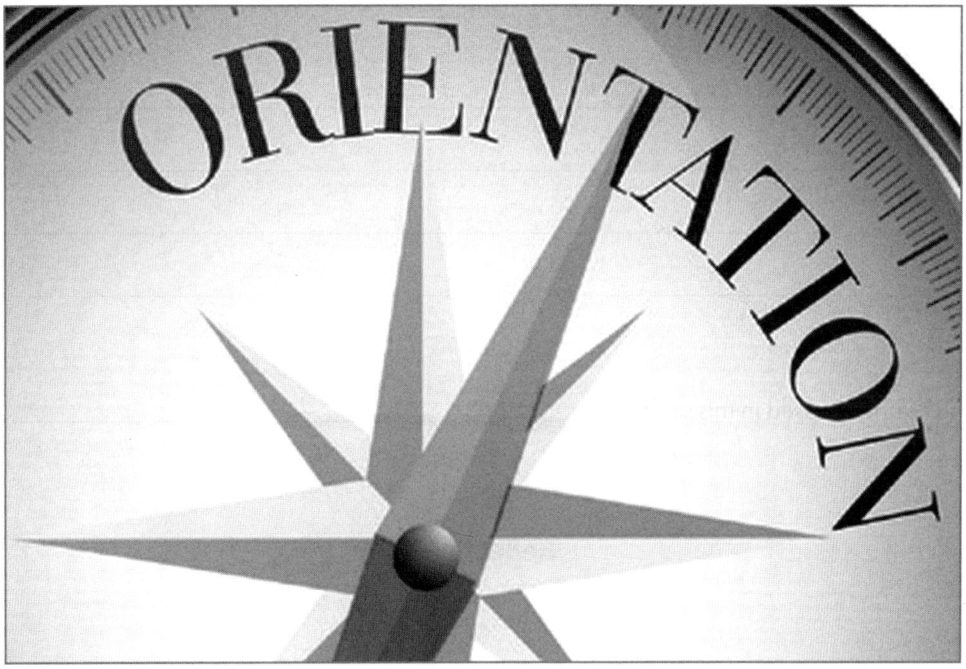

Session: 1

Name(s) of the faculty: ____________________

Date: ____________________ Time: ____________________ to ____________________

Duration: ____________________

Learning objective(s) of the session (Write from the presentation or as instructed by the faculty):

1. ____________________
2. ____________________
3. ____________________
4. ____________________

Teaching learning method(s) used in this session: ____________________

Reflections

1. Please describe what happened during the session:

____

____

2. What did you learn in this session?

____

____

3. How do you think what you learnt in this session will be useful for you?

____

____

____

____

Signature of the Teacher Domain: K/A/S/C Level Attained: K/KH/SH/P

Session: 2

Name(s) of the faculty: ______________________________

Date: ____________________ Time: ______________ to ______________

Duration: ____________________

Learning objective(s) of the session (Write from the presentation or as instructed by the faculty):

1. ______________________________
2. ______________________________
3. ______________________________
4. ______________________________

Teaching learning method(s) used in this session: ______________________________

Reflections

1. Please describe what happened during the session:

____

____

2. What did you learn in this session?

____

____

3. How do you think what you learnt in this session will be useful for you?

____

____

____

____

Signature of the Teacher Domain: K/A/S/C Level Attained: K/KH/SH/P

Session: 3

Name(s) of the faculty: ______________________________

Date: ____________________ Time: ______________ to ______________

Duration: ____________________

Learning objective(s) of the session (Write from the presentation or as instructed by the faculty):

1. ______________________________
2. ______________________________
3. ______________________________
4. ______________________________

Teaching learning method(s) used in this session: ______________________________

Reflections

1. Please describe what happened during the session:

____

____

2. What did you learn in this session?

____

____

3. How do you think what you learnt in this session will be useful for you?

____

____

____

____

Signature of the Teacher Domain: K/A/S/C Level Attained: K/KH/SH/P

Session: 4

Name(s) of the faculty: ____________________

Date: ____________________ Time: ____________ to ____________

Duration: ____________________

Learning objective(s) of the session (Write from the presentation or as instructed by the faculty):

1. ____________________
2. ____________________
3. ____________________
4. ____________________

Teaching learning method(s) used in this session: ____________________

Reflections

1. Please describe what happened during the session:

____

____

2. What did you learn in this session?

____

____

3. How do you think what you learnt in this session will be useful for you?

____

____

____

____

Signature of the Teacher Domain: K/A/S/C Level Attained: K/KH/SH/P

Session: 5

Name(s) of the faculty: ____________________

Date: ____________________ Time: ____________ to ____________

Duration: ____________________

Learning objective(s) of the session (Write from the presentation or as instructed by the faculty):

1. ____________________
2. ____________________
3. ____________________
4. ____________________

Teaching learning method(s) used in this session: ____________________

Reflections

1. Please describe what happened during the session:

____

____

2. What did you learn in this session?

____

____

3. How do you think what you learnt in this session will be useful for you?

____

____

____

____

Signature of the Teacher Domain: K/A/S/C Level Attained: K/KH/SH/P

Session: 6

Name(s) of the faculty: ____________________

Date: ____________________ Time: ____________ to ____________

Duration: ____________________

Learning objective(s) of the session (Write from the presentation or as instructed by the faculty):

1. ____________________
2. ____________________
3. ____________________
4. ____________________

Teaching learning method(s) used in this session: ____________________

Reflections

1. Please describe what happened during the session:

____

____

2. What did you learn in this session?

____

____

3. How do you think what you learnt in this session will be useful for you?

____

____

____

____

Signature of the Teacher Domain: K/A/S/C Level Attained: K/KH/SH/P

Session: 7

Name(s) of the faculty: ______________________________

Date: ____________________ Time: ______________ to ______________

Duration: ____________________

Learning objective(s) of the session (Write from the presentation or as instructed by the faculty):

1. ______________________________
2. ______________________________
3. ______________________________
4. ______________________________

Teaching learning method(s) used in this session: ______________________________

Reflections

1. Please describe what happened during the session:

____
____

2. What did you learn in this session?

____
____

3. How do you think what you learnt in this session will be useful for you?

____
____
____
____

Signature of the Teacher Domain: K/A/S/C Level Attained: K/KH/SH/P

Session: 8

Name(s) of the faculty: ______________________________

Date: ____________________ Time: ______________ to ______________

Duration: ____________________

Learning objective(s) of the session (Write from the presentation or as instructed by the faculty):

1. ______________________________
2. ______________________________
3. ______________________________
4. ______________________________

Teaching learning method(s) used in this session: ______________________________

Reflections

1. Please describe what happened during the session:

____

____

2. What did you learn in this session?

____

____

3. How do you think what you learnt in this session will be useful for you?

____

____

____

____

Signature of the Teacher Domain: K/A/S/C Level Attained: K/KH/SH/P

Session: 9

Name(s) of the faculty: ______________________________

Date: ______________________ Time: ______________ to ______________

Duration: ______________________

Learning objective(s) of the session (Write from the presentation or as instructed by the faculty):

1. ______________________________

2. ______________________________

3. ______________________________

4. ______________________________

Teaching learning method(s) used in this session: ______________________________

Reflections

1. Please describe what happened during the session:

____

____

2. What did you learn in this session?

____

____

3. How do you think what you learnt in this session will be useful for you?

____

____

____

____

Signature of the Teacher Domain: K/A/S/C Level Attained: K/KH/SH/P

Session: 10

Name(s) of the faculty: ______________________________

Date: ____________________ Time: ______________ to ______________

Duration: ____________________

Learning objective(s) of the session (Write from the presentation or as instructed by the faculty):

1. ______________________________
2. ______________________________
3. ______________________________
4. ______________________________

Teaching learning method(s) used in this session: ______________________________

Reflections

1. Please describe what happened during the session:

____

____

2. What did you learn in this session?

____

____

3. How do you think what you learnt in this session will be useful for you?

____

____

____

____

Signature of the Teacher Domain: K/A/S/C Level Attained: K/KH/SH/P

Session: 11

Name(s) of the faculty: ___________________________________

Date: ____________________ Time: ____________ to ____________

Duration: ____________________

Learning objective(s) of the session (Write from the presentation or as instructed by the faculty):

1. ___________________________________
2. ___________________________________
3. ___________________________________
4. ___________________________________

Teaching learning method(s) used in this session: ___________________________________

Reflections

1. Please describe what happened during the session:

____

____

2. What did you learn in this session?

____

____

3. How do you think what you learnt in this session will be useful for you?

____

____

____

____

Signature of the Teacher Domain: K/A/S/C Level Attained: K/KH/SH/P

Session: 12

Name(s) of the faculty: ______________________

Date: ______________________ Time: ______________ to ______________

Duration: ______________________

Learning objective(s) of the session (Write from the presentation or as instructed by the faculty):

1. ______________________
2. ______________________
3. ______________________
4. ______________________

Teaching learning method(s) used in this session: ______________________

Reflections

1. Please describe what happened during the session:

____

____

2. What did you learn in this session?

____

____

3. How do you think what you learnt in this session will be useful for you?

____

____

____

____

Signature of the Teacher Domain: K/A/S/C Level Attained: K/KH/SH/P

Session: 13

Name(s) of the faculty: ______________________________

Date: ____________________ Time: ____________ to ____________

Duration: ____________________

Learning objective(s) of the session (Write from the presentation or as instructed by the faculty):

1. ______________________________
2. ______________________________
3. ______________________________
4. ______________________________

Teaching learning method(s) used in this session: ______________________________

Reflections

1. Please describe what happened during the session:

____

____

2. What did you learn in this session?

____

____

3. How do you think what you learnt in this session will be useful for you?

____

____

____

____

Signature of the Teacher Domain: K/A/S/C Level Attained: K/KH/SH/P

Session: 14

Name(s) of the faculty: ______________________________

Date: ____________________ Time: ______________ to ______________

Duration: ____________________

Learning objective(s) of the session (Write from the presentation or as instructed by the faculty):

1. ______________________________
2. ______________________________
3. ______________________________
4. ______________________________

Teaching learning method(s) used in this session: ______________________________

Reflections

1. Please describe what happened during the session:

____

____

2. What did you learn in this session?

____

____

3. How do you think what you learnt in this session will be useful for you?

____

____

____

____

Signature of the Teacher Domain: K/A/S/C Level Attained: K/KH/SH/P

Session: 15

Name(s) of the faculty: ______________________________

Date: ____________________ Time: ______________ to ______________

Duration: ____________________

Learning objective(s) of the session (Write from the presentation or as instructed by the faculty):

1. ______________________________
2. ______________________________
3. ______________________________
4. ______________________________

Teaching learning method(s) used in this session: ______________________________

Reflections

1. Please describe what happened during the session:

____

____

2. What did you learn in this session?

____

____

3. How do you think what you learnt in this session will be useful for you?

____

____

____

____

Signature of the Teacher Domain: K/A/S/C Level Attained: K/KH/SH/P

Session: 16

Name(s) of the faculty: ______________________________

Date: ____________________ Time: ______________ to ______________

Duration: ____________________

Learning objective(s) of the session (Write from the presentation or as instructed by the faculty):

1. ______________________________
2. ______________________________
3. ______________________________
4. ______________________________

Teaching learning method(s) used in this session: ______________________________

Reflections

1. Please describe what happened during the session:

____

____

2. What did you learn in this session?

____

____

3. How do you think what you learnt in this session will be useful for you?

____

____

____

____

Signature of the Teacher Domain: K/A/S/C Level Attained: K/KH/SH/P

Session: 17

Name(s) of the faculty: ______________________________

Date: ____________________ Time: ____________ to ____________

Duration: ____________________

Learning objective(s) of the session (Write from the presentation or as instructed by the faculty):

1. ______________________________
2. ______________________________
3. ______________________________
4. ______________________________

Teaching learning method(s) used in this session: ______________________________

Reflections

1. Please describe what happened during the session:

____

____

2. What did you learn in this session?

____

____

3. How do you think what you learnt in this session will be useful for you?

____

____

____

____

Signature of the Teacher Domain: K/A/S/C Level Attained: K/KH/SH/P

Session: 18

Name(s) of the faculty: ____________________

Date: ____________________ Time: ____________ to ____________

Duration: ____________________

Learning objective(s) of the session (Write from the presentation or as instructed by the faculty):

1. ____________________
2. ____________________
3. ____________________
4. ____________________

Teaching learning method(s) used in this session: ____________________

Reflections

1. Please describe what happened during the session:

____

____

2. What did you learn in this session?

____

____

3. How do you think what you learnt in this session will be useful for you?

____

____

____

____

Signature of the Teacher Domain: K/A/S/C Level Attained: K/KH/SH/P

Session: 19

Name(s) of the faculty: ______________________________

Date: ____________________ Time: ______________ to ______________

Duration: ____________________

Learning objective(s) of the session (Write from the presentation or as instructed by the faculty):

1. ______________________________
2. ______________________________
3. ______________________________
4. ______________________________

Teaching learning method(s) used in this session: ______________________________

Reflections

1. Please describe what happened during the session:

____

____

2. What did you learn in this session?

____

____

3. How do you think what you learnt in this session will be useful for you?

____

____

____

____

Signature of the Teacher Domain: K/A/S/C Level Attained: K/KH/SH/P

Session: 20

Name(s) of the faculty: ____________________

Date: ____________________ Time: ____________ to ____________

Duration: ____________________

Learning objective(s) of the session (Write from the presentation or as instructed by the faculty):

1. ____________________
2. ____________________
3. ____________________
4. ____________________

Teaching learning method(s) used in this session: ____________________

Reflections

1. Please describe what happened during the session:

____

____

2. What did you learn in this session?

____

____

3. How do you think what you learnt in this session will be useful for you?

____

____

____

____

Signature of the Teacher Domain: K/A/S/C Level Attained: K/KH/SH/P

Session: 21

Name(s) of the faculty: ______________________________

Date: ____________________ Time: ______________ to ______________

Duration: ____________________

Learning objective(s) of the session (Write from the presentation or as instructed by the faculty):

1. ______________________________
2. ______________________________
3. ______________________________
4. ______________________________

Teaching learning method(s) used in this session: ______________________________

Reflections

1. Please describe what happened during the session:

____

____

2. What did you learn in this session?

____

____

3. How do you think what you learnt in this session will be useful for you?

____

____

____

____

Signature of the Teacher Domain: K/A/S/C Level Attained: K/KH/SH/P

Session: 22

Name(s) of the faculty: ______________________________

Date: ____________________ Time: ______________ to ______________

Duration: ____________________

Learning objective(s) of the session (Write from the presentation or as instructed by the faculty):

1. ______________________________
2. ______________________________
3. ______________________________
4. ______________________________

Teaching learning method(s) used in this session: ______________________________

Reflections

1. Please describe what happened during the session:

____

____

2. What did you learn in this session?

____

____

3. How do you think what you learnt in this session will be useful for you?

____

____

____

____

Signature of the Teacher Domain: K/A/S/C Level Attained: K/KH/SH/P

Session: 23

Name(s) of the faculty: ______________________________

Date: ____________________ Time: ______________ to ______________

Duration: ____________________

Learning objective(s) of the session (Write from the presentation or as instructed by the faculty):

1. ______________________________
2. ______________________________
3. ______________________________
4. ______________________________

Teaching learning method(s) used in this session: ______________________________

Reflections

1. Please describe what happened during the session:

____

____

2. What did you learn in this session?

____

____

3. How do you think what you learnt in this session will be useful for you?

____

____

____

____

Signature of the Teacher Domain: K/A/S/C Level Attained: K/KH/SH/P

Session: 24

Name(s) of the faculty: ______________________________

Date: ____________________ Time: ______________ to ______________

Duration: ____________________

Learning objective(s) of the session (Write from the presentation or as instructed by the faculty):

1. ______________________________
2. ______________________________
3. ______________________________
4. ______________________________

Teaching learning method(s) used in this session: ______________________________

Reflections

1. Please describe what happened during the session:

____

____

2. What did you learn in this session?

____

____

3. How do you think what you learnt in this session will be useful for you?

____

____

____

____

Signature of the Teacher Domain: K/A/S/C Level Attained: K/KH/SH/P

Session: 25

Name(s) of the faculty: ______________________________

Date: ____________________ Time: ______________ to ______________

Duration: ____________________

Learning objective(s) of the session (Write from the presentation or as instructed by the faculty):

1. ______________________________
2. ______________________________
3. ______________________________
4. ______________________________

Teaching learning method(s) used in this session: ______________________________

Reflections

1. Please describe what happened during the session:

____

____

2. What did you learn in this session?

____

____

3. How do you think what you learnt in this session will be useful for you?

____

____

____

____

Signature of the Teacher Domain: K/A/S/C Level Attained: K/KH/SH/P

Session: 26

Name(s) of the faculty: ______________________________

Date: ____________________ Time: ______________ to ______________

Duration: ____________________

Learning objective(s) of the session (Write from the presentation or as instructed by the faculty):

1. ______________________________
2. ______________________________
3. ______________________________
4. ______________________________

Teaching learning method(s) used in this session: ______________________________

Reflections

1. Please describe what happened during the session:

____

____

2. What did you learn in this session?

____

____

3. How do you think what you learnt in this session will be useful for you?

____

____

____

____

Signature of the Teacher Domain: K/A/S/C Level Attained: K/KH/SH/P

Session: 27

Name(s) of the faculty: ______________________________

Date: ____________________ Time: ______________ to ______________

Duration: ____________________

Learning objective(s) of the session (Write from the presentation or as instructed by the faculty):

1. ______________________________
2. ______________________________
3. ______________________________
4. ______________________________

Teaching learning method(s) used in this session: ______________________________

Reflections

1. Please describe what happened during the session:

____

____

2. What did you learn in this session?

____

____

3. How do you think what you learnt in this session will be useful for you?

____

____

____

____

Signature of the Teacher Domain: K/A/S/C Level Attained: K/KH/SH/P

Session: 28

Name(s) of the faculty: ____________________

Date: ____________________ Time: ____________ to ____________

Duration: ____________________

Learning objective(s) of the session (Write from the presentation or as instructed by the faculty):

1. ____________________
2. ____________________
3. ____________________
4. ____________________

Teaching learning method(s) used in this session: ____________________

Reflections

1. Please describe what happened during the session:

____

____

2. What did you learn in this session?

____

____

3. How do you think what you learnt in this session will be useful for you?

____

____

____

____

Signature of the Teacher Domain: K/A/S/C Level Attained: K/KH/SH/P

Session: 29

Name(s) of the faculty: ____________________

Date: ____________________ Time: __________ to __________

Duration: ____________________

Learning objective(s) of the session (Write from the presentation or as instructed by the faculty):

1. ____________________
2. ____________________
3. ____________________
4. ____________________

Teaching learning method(s) used in this session: ____________________

Reflections

1. Please describe what happened during the session:

____

____

2. What did you learn in this session?

____

____

3. How do you think what you learnt in this session will be useful for you?

____

____

____

____

Signature of the Teacher Domain: K/A/S/C Level Attained: K/KH/SH/P

Session: 30

Name(s) of the faculty: ____________________

Date: ____________________ Time: ____________ to ____________

Duration: ____________________

Learning objective(s) of the session (Write from the presentation or as instructed by the faculty):

1. ____________________
2. ____________________
3. ____________________
4. ____________________

Teaching learning method(s) used in this session: ____________________

Reflections

1. Please describe what happened during the session:

____

____

2. What did you learn in this session?

____

____

3. How do you think what you learnt in this session will be useful for you?

____

____

____

____

Signature of the Teacher Domain: K/A/S/C Level Attained: K/KH/SH/P

Skills Module

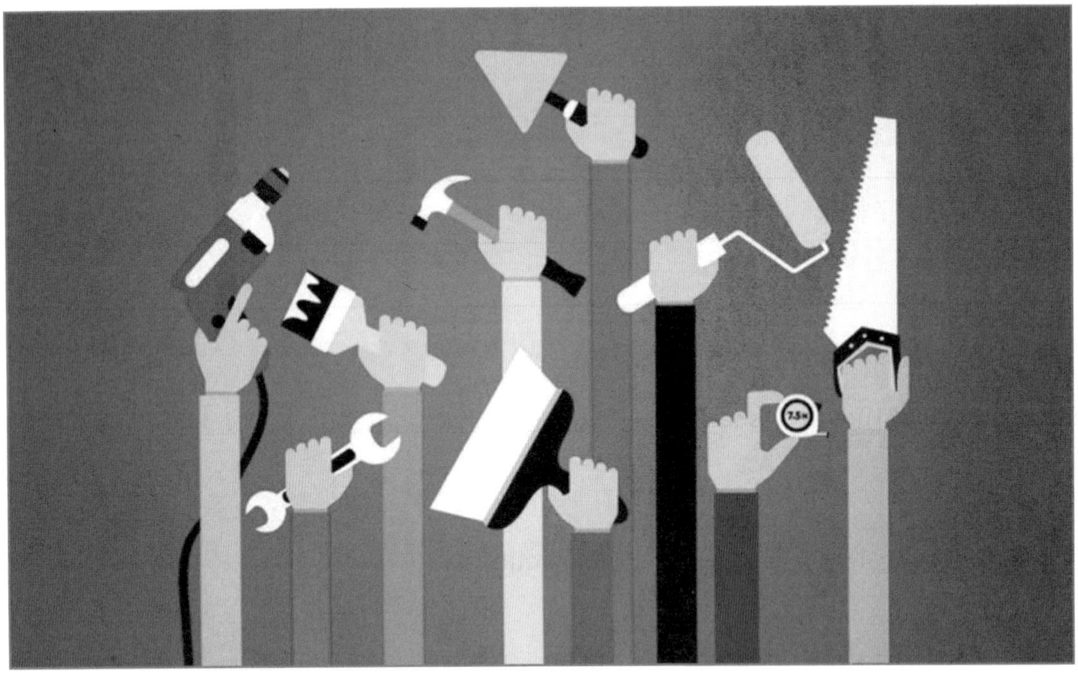

Session: 1

Name(s) of the faculty: ______________________________

Date: ____________________ Time: ____________ to ____________

Duration: ____________________

Learning objective(s) of the session (Write from the presentation or as instructed by the faculty):

1. ______________________________
2. ______________________________
3. ______________________________
4. ______________________________

Teaching learning method(s) used in this session: ______________________________

Reflections

1. Please describe what happened during the session:

____

____

2. What did you learn in this session?

____

____

3. How do you think what you learnt in this session will be useful for you?

____

____

____

____

Signature of the Teacher Domain: K/A/S/C Level Attained: K/KH/SH/P

Session: 2

Name(s) of the faculty: ____________________

Date: ____________________ Time: ____________ to ____________

Duration: ____________________

Learning objective(s) of the session (Write from the presentation or as instructed by the faculty):

1. ____________________
2. ____________________
3. ____________________
4. ____________________

Teaching learning method(s) used in this session: ____________________

Reflections

1. Please describe what happened during the session:

____

____

2. What did you learn in this session?

____

____

3. How do you think what you learnt in this session will be useful for you?

____

____

____

____

Signature of the Teacher Domain: K/A/S/C Level Attained: K/KH/SH/P

Session: 3

Name(s) of the faculty: ______________________________

Date: ____________________ Time: ____________ to ____________

Duration: ____________________

Learning objective(s) of the session (Write from the presentation or as instructed by the faculty):

1. ______________________________
2. ______________________________
3. ______________________________
4. ______________________________

Teaching learning method(s) used in this session: ______________________________

Reflections

1. Please describe what happened during the session:

____

____

2. What did you learn in this session?

____

____

3. How do you think what you learnt in this session will be useful for you?

____

____

____

____

Signature of the Teacher Domain: K/A/S/C Level Attained: K/KH/SH/P

Session: 4

Name(s) of the faculty: ____________________

Date: ____________________ Time: ____________ to ____________

Duration: ____________________

Learning objective(s) of the session (Write from the presentation or as instructed by the faculty):

1. ____________________
2. ____________________
3. ____________________
4. ____________________

Teaching learning method(s) used in this session: ____________________

Reflections

1. Please describe what happened during the session:

____

____

2. What did you learn in this session?

____

____

3. How do you think what you learnt in this session will be useful for you?

____

____

____

____

Signature of the Teacher Domain: K/A/S/C Level Attained: K/KH/SH/P

Session: 5

Name(s) of the faculty: ____________________

Date: ____________________ Time: ____________ to ____________

Duration: ____________________

Learning objective(s) of the session (Write from the presentation or as instructed by the faculty):

1. ____________________
2. ____________________
3. ____________________
4. ____________________

Teaching learning method(s) used in this session: ____________________

Reflections

1. Please describe what happened during the session:

____

____

2. What did you learn in this session?

____

____

3. How do you think what you learnt in this session will be useful for you?

____

____

____

____

Signature of the Teacher Domain: K/A/S/C Level Attained: K/KH/SH/P

Session: 6

Name(s) of the faculty: ____________________

Date: ____________________ Time: ____________ to ____________

Duration: ____________________

Learning objective(s) of the session (Write from the presentation or as instructed by the faculty):

1. ____________________
2. ____________________
3. ____________________
4. ____________________

Teaching learning method(s) used in this session: ____________________

Reflections

1. Please describe what happened during the session:

____

____

2. What did you learn in this session?

____

____

3. How do you think what you learnt in this session will be useful for you?

____

____

____

____

Signature of the Teacher Domain: K/A/S/C Level Attained: K/KH/SH/P

Session: 7

Name(s) of the faculty: ____________________

Date: ____________________ Time: ____________ to ____________

Duration: ____________________

Learning objective(s) of the session (Write from the presentation or as instructed by the faculty):

1. ____________________
2. ____________________
3. ____________________
4. ____________________

Teaching learning method(s) used in this session: ____________________

Reflections

1. Please describe what happened during the session:

____

____

2. What did you learn in this session?

____

____

3. How do you think what you learnt in this session will be useful for you?

____

____

____

____

Signature of the Teacher Domain: K/A/S/C Level Attained: K/KH/SH/P

Session: 8

Name(s) of the faculty: ____________________

Date: ____________________ Time: ____________ to ____________

Duration: ____________________

Learning objective(s) of the session (Write from the presentation or as instructed by the faculty):

1. ____________________
2. ____________________
3. ____________________
4. ____________________

Teaching learning method(s) used in this session: ____________________

Reflections

1. Please describe what happened during the session:

____

____

2. What did you learn in this session?

____

____

3. How do you think what you learnt in this session will be useful for you?

____

____

____

____

Signature of the Teacher Domain: K/A/S/C Level Attained: K/KH/SH/P

Session: 9

Name(s) of the faculty: ____________________

Date: ____________________ Time: __________ to __________

Duration: ____________________

Learning objective(s) of the session (Write from the presentation or as instructed by the faculty):

1. ____________________
2. ____________________
3. ____________________
4. ____________________

Teaching learning method(s) used in this session: ____________________

Reflections

1. Please describe what happened during the session:

____

____

2. What did you learn in this session?

____

____

3. How do you think what you learnt in this session will be useful for you?

____

____

____

____

Signature of the Teacher Domain: K/A/S/C Level Attained: K/KH/SH/P

Session: 10

Name(s) of the faculty: ____________________

Date: ____________________ Time: ____________ to ____________

Duration: ____________________

Learning objective(s) of the session (Write from the presentation or as instructed by the faculty):

1. ____________________
2. ____________________
3. ____________________
4. ____________________

Teaching learning method(s) used in this session: ____________________

Reflections

1. Please describe what happened during the session:

____

____

2. What did you learn in this session?

____

____

3. How do you think what you learnt in this session will be useful for you?

____

____

____

____

Signature of the Teacher Domain: K/A/S/C Level Attained: K/KH/SH/P

Session: 11

Name(s) of the faculty: ____________________

Date: ____________________ Time: ____________ to ____________

Duration: ____________________

Learning objective(s) of the session (Write from the presentation or as instructed by the faculty):

1. ____________________
2. ____________________
3. ____________________
4. ____________________

Teaching learning method(s) used in this session: ____________________

Reflections

1. Please describe what happened during the session:

____

____

2. What did you learn in this session?

____

____

3. How do you think what you learnt in this session will be useful for you?

____

____

____

____

Signature of the Teacher Domain: K/A/S/C Level Attained: K/KH/SH/P

Session: 12

Name(s) of the faculty: ____________________

Date: ____________________ Time: ____________ to ____________

Duration: ____________________

Learning objective(s) of the session (Write from the presentation or as instructed by the faculty):

1. ____________________
2. ____________________
3. ____________________
4. ____________________

Teaching learning method(s) used in this session: ____________________

Reflections

1. Please describe what happened during the session:

____

____

2. What did you learn in this session?

____

____

3. How do you think what you learnt in this session will be useful for you?

____

____

____

____

Signature of the Teacher Domain: K/A/S/C Level Attained: K/KH/SH/P

Session: 13

Name(s) of the faculty: ____________________

Date: ____________________ Time: ____________ to ____________

Duration: ____________________

Learning objective(s) of the session (Write from the presentation or as instructed by the faculty):

1. ____________________
2. ____________________
3. ____________________
4. ____________________

Teaching learning method(s) used in this session: ____________________

Reflections

1. Please describe what happened during the session:

____

2. What did you learn in this session?

____

3. How do you think what you learnt in this session will be useful for you?

____

Signature of the Teacher Domain: K/A/S/C Level Attained: K/KH/SH/P

Session: 14

Name(s) of the faculty: ______________________________

Date: ____________________ Time: ____________ to ____________

Duration: ____________________

Learning objective(s) of the session (Write from the presentation or as instructed by the faculty):

1. ______________________________
2. ______________________________
3. ______________________________
4. ______________________________

Teaching learning method(s) used in this session: ______________________________

Reflections

1. Please describe what happened during the session:

____

____

2. What did you learn in this session?

____

____

3. How do you think what you learnt in this session will be useful for you?

____

____

____

____

Signature of the Teacher Domain: K/A/S/C Level Attained: K/KH/SH/P

Session: 15

Name(s) of the faculty: ______________________________

Date: ____________________ Time: ____________ to ____________

Duration: ____________________

Learning objective(s) of the session (Write from the presentation or as instructed by the faculty):

1. ______________________________
2. ______________________________
3. ______________________________
4. ______________________________

Teaching learning method(s) used in this session: ______________________________

Reflections

1. Please describe what happened during the session:

____

____

2. What did you learn in this session?

____

____

3. How do you think what you learnt in this session will be useful for you?

____

____

____

____

Signature of the Teacher Domain: K/A/S/C Level Attained: K/KH/SH/P

Session: 16

Name(s) of the faculty: ____________________

Date: ____________________ Time: ____________ to ____________

Duration: ____________________

Learning objective(s) of the session (Write from the presentation or as instructed by the faculty):

1. ____________________
2. ____________________
3. ____________________
4. ____________________

Teaching learning method(s) used in this session: ____________________

Reflections

1. Please describe what happened during the session:

____

____

2. What did you learn in this session?

____

____

3. How do you think what you learnt in this session will be useful for you?

____

____

____

____

Signature of the Teacher Domain: K/A/S/C Level Attained: K/KH/SH/P

Session: 17

Name(s) of the faculty: ____________________

Date: ____________________ Time: __________ to __________

Duration: ____________________

Learning objective(s) of the session (Write from the presentation or as instructed by the faculty):

1. ____________________
2. ____________________
3. ____________________
4. ____________________

Teaching learning method(s) used in this session: ____________________

Reflections

1. Please describe what happened during the session:

____

____

2. What did you learn in this session?

____

____

3. How do you think what you learnt in this session will be useful for you?

____

____

____

____

Signature of the Teacher Domain: K/A/S/C Level Attained: K/KH/SH/P

Session: 18

Name(s) of the faculty: ____________________

Date: ____________________ Time: ____________ to ____________

Duration: ____________________

Learning objective(s) of the session (Write from the presentation or as instructed by the faculty):

1. ____________________
2. ____________________
3. ____________________
4. ____________________

Teaching learning method(s) used in this session: ____________________

Reflections

1. Please describe what happened during the session:

____

____

2. What did you learn in this session?

____

____

3. How do you think what you learnt in this session will be useful for you?

____

____

____

____

Signature of the Teacher Domain: K/A/S/C Level Attained: K/KH/SH/P

Session: 19

Name(s) of the faculty: ____________________

Date: ____________________ Time: ____________ to ____________

Duration: ____________________

Learning objective(s) of the session (Write from the presentation or as instructed by the faculty):

1. ____________________
2. ____________________
3. ____________________
4. ____________________

Teaching learning method(s) used in this session: ____________________

Reflections

1. Please describe what happened during the session:

____

____

2. What did you learn in this session?

____

____

3. How do you think what you learnt in this session will be useful for you?

____

____

____

____

Signature of the Teacher Domain: K/A/S/C Level Attained: K/KH/SH/P

Session: 20

Name(s) of the faculty: ____________________

Date: ____________________ Time: ____________ to ____________

Duration: ____________________

Learning objective(s) of the session (Write from the presentation or as instructed by the faculty):

1. ____________________
2. ____________________
3. ____________________
4. ____________________

Teaching learning method(s) used in this session: ____________________

Reflections

1. Please describe what happened during the session:

____

____

2. What did you learn in this session?

____

____

3. How do you think what you learnt in this session will be useful for you?

____

____

____

____

Signature of the Teacher Domain: K/A/S/C Level Attained: K/KH/SH/P

Session: 21

Name(s) of the faculty: ____________________

Date: ____________________ Time: ____________ to ____________

Duration: ____________________

Learning objective(s) of the session (Write from the presentation or as instructed by the faculty):

1. ____________________
2. ____________________
3. ____________________
4. ____________________

Teaching learning method(s) used in this session: ____________________

Reflections

1. Please describe what happened during the session:

____

____

2. What did you learn in this session?

____

____

3. How do you think what you learnt in this session will be useful for you?

____

____

____

____

Signature of the Teacher Domain: K/A/S/C Level Attained: K/KH/SH/P

Session: 22

Name(s) of the faculty: ____________________

Date: ____________________ Time: ____________ to ____________

Duration: ____________________

Learning objective(s) of the session (Write from the presentation or as instructed by the faculty):

1. ____________________
2. ____________________
3. ____________________
4. ____________________

Teaching learning method(s) used in this session: ____________________

Reflections

1. Please describe what happened during the session:

____

____

2. What did you learn in this session?

____

____

3. How do you think what you learnt in this session will be useful for you?

____

____

____

____

Signature of the Teacher Domain: K/A/S/C Level Attained: K/KH/SH/P

Session: 23

Name(s) of the faculty: ____________________

Date: ____________________ Time: ____________ to ____________

Duration: ____________________

Learning objective(s) of the session (Write from the presentation or as instructed by the faculty):

1. ____________________
2. ____________________
3. ____________________
4. ____________________

Teaching learning method(s) used in this session: ____________________

Reflections

1. Please describe what happened during the session:

____

____

2. What did you learn in this session?

____

____

3. How do you think what you learnt in this session will be useful for you?

____

____

____

____

Signature of the Teacher Domain: K/A/S/C Level Attained: K/KH/SH/P

Session: 24

Name(s) of the faculty: ____________________

Date: ____________________ Time: ____________ to ____________

Duration: ____________________

Learning objective(s) of the session (Write from the presentation or as instructed by the faculty):

1. ____________________
2. ____________________
3. ____________________
4. ____________________

Teaching learning method(s) used in this session: ____________________

Reflections

1. Please describe what happened during the session:

____

____

2. What did you learn in this session?

____

____

3. How do you think what you learnt in this session will be useful for you?

____

____

____

____

Signature of the Teacher Domain: K/A/S/C Level Attained: K/KH/SH/P

Session: 25

Name(s) of the faculty: ____________________

Date: ____________________ Time: ____________ to ____________

Duration: ____________________

Learning objective(s) of the session (Write from the presentation or as instructed by the faculty):

1. ____________________
2. ____________________
3. ____________________
4. ____________________

Teaching learning method(s) used in this session: ____________________

Reflections

1. Please describe what happened during the session:

____

____

2. What did you learn in this session?

____

____

3. How do you think what you learnt in this session will be useful for you?

____

____

____

____

Signature of the Teacher Domain: K/A/S/C Level Attained: K/KH/SH/P

Session: 26

Name(s) of the faculty: ______________________________

Date: ____________________ Time: ____________ to ____________

Duration: ____________________

Learning objective(s) of the session (Write from the presentation or as instructed by the faculty):

1. ______________________________
2. ______________________________
3. ______________________________
4. ______________________________

Teaching learning method(s) used in this session: ______________________________

Reflections

1. Please describe what happened during the session:

____

____

2. What did you learn in this session?

____

____

3. How do you think what you learnt in this session will be useful for you?

____

____

____

____

Signature of the Teacher Domain: K/A/S/C Level Attained: K/KH/SH/P

Session: 27

Name(s) of the faculty: ____________________

Date: ____________________ Time: ____________ to ____________

Duration: ____________________

Learning objective(s) of the session (Write from the presentation or as instructed by the faculty):

1. ____________________
2. ____________________
3. ____________________
4. ____________________

Teaching learning method(s) used in this session: ____________________

Reflections

1. Please describe what happened during the session:

____

____

2. What did you learn in this session?

____

____

3. How do you think what you learnt in this session will be useful for you?

____

____

____

____

Signature of the Teacher Domain: K/A/S/C Level Attained: K/KH/SH/P

Session: 28

Name(s) of the faculty: ______________________________

Date: ____________________ Time: ______________ to ______________

Duration: ____________________

Learning objective(s) of the session (Write from the presentation or as instructed by the faculty):

1. ______________________________
2. ______________________________
3. ______________________________
4. ______________________________

Teaching learning method(s) used in this session: ______________________________

Reflections

1. Please describe what happened during the session:

____

____

2. What did you learn in this session?

____

____

3. How do you think what you learnt in this session will be useful for you?

____

____

____

____

Signature of the Teacher Domain: K/A/S/C Level Attained: K/KH/SH/P

Session: 29

Name(s) of the faculty: ____________________

Date: ____________________ Time: ____________ to ____________

Duration: ____________________

Learning objective(s) of the session (Write from the presentation or as instructed by the faculty):

1. ____________________
2. ____________________
3. ____________________
4. ____________________

Teaching learning method(s) used in this session: ____________________

Reflections

1. Please describe what happened during the session:

____

____

2. What did you learn in this session?

____

____

3. How do you think what you learnt in this session will be useful for you?

____

____

____

____

Signature of the Teacher Domain: K/A/S/C Level Attained: K/KH/SH/P

Session: 30

Name(s) of the faculty: ____________________

Date: ____________________ Time: ____________ to ____________

Duration: ____________________

Learning objective(s) of the session (Write from the presentation or as instructed by the faculty):

1. ____________________
2. ____________________
3. ____________________
4. ____________________

Teaching learning method(s) used in this session: ____________________

Reflections

1. Please describe what happened during the session:

____

____

2. What did you learn in this session?

____

____

3. How do you think what you learnt in this session will be useful for you?

____

____

____

____

Signature of the Teacher Domain: K/A/S/C Level Attained: K/KH/SH/P

Community Orientation Module

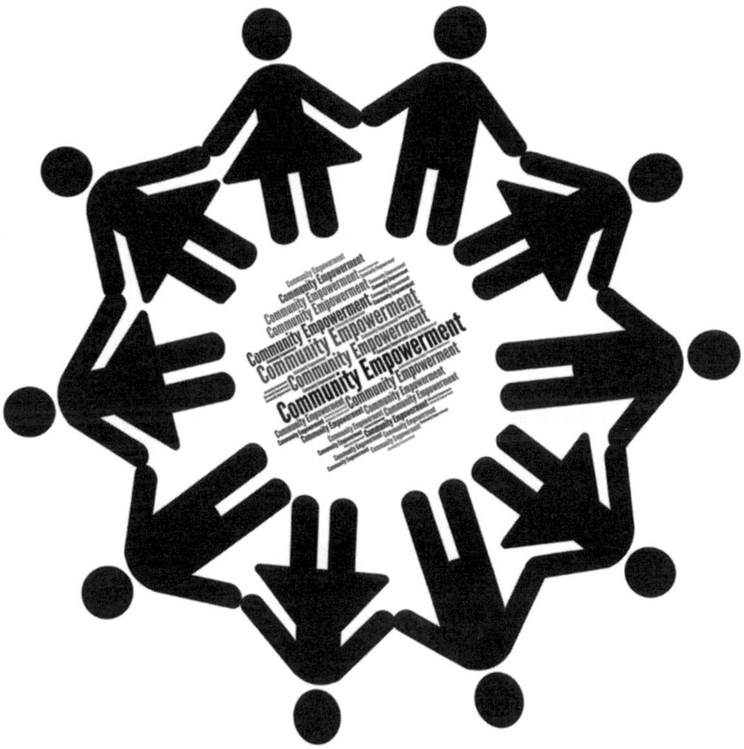

Session: 1

Name(s) of the faculty: ____________________

Date: ____________________ Time: ____________ to ____________

Duration: ____________________

Learning objective(s) of the session (Write from the presentation or as instructed by the faculty):

1. ____________________
2. ____________________
3. ____________________
4. ____________________

Teaching learning method(s) used in this session: ____________________

Reflections

1. Please describe what happened during the session:

____

____

2. What did you learn in this session?

____

____

3. How do you think what you learnt in this session will be useful for you?

____

____

____

____

Signature of the Teacher Domain: K/A/S/C Level Attained: K/KH/SH/P

Session: 2

Name(s) of the faculty: ____________________

Date: ____________________ Time: ____________ to ____________

Duration: ____________________

Learning objective(s) of the session (Write from the presentation or as instructed by the faculty):

1. ____________________
2. ____________________
3. ____________________
4. ____________________

Teaching learning method(s) used in this session: ____________________

Reflections

1. Please describe what happened during the session:

____

____

2. What did you learn in this session?

____

____

3. How do you think what you learnt in this session will be useful for you?

____

____

____

____

Signature of the Teacher Domain: K/A/S/C Level Attained: K/KH/SH/P

Session: 3

Name(s) of the faculty: ____________________

Date: ____________________ Time: __________ to __________

Duration: ____________________

Learning objective(s) of the session (Write from the presentation or as instructed by the faculty):

1. ____________________
2. ____________________
3. ____________________
4. ____________________

Teaching learning method(s) used in this session: ____________________

Reflections

1. Please describe what happened during the session:

____

____

2. What did you learn in this session?

____

____

3. How do you think what you learnt in this session will be useful for you?

____

____

____

____

Signature of the Teacher Domain: K/A/S/C Level Attained: K/KH/SH/P

Session: 4

Name(s) of the faculty: ____________________

Date: ____________________ Time: ____________ to ____________

Duration: ____________________

Learning objective(s) of the session (Write from the presentation or as instructed by the faculty):

1. ____________________
2. ____________________
3. ____________________
4. ____________________

Teaching learning method(s) used in this session: ____________________

Reflections

1. Please describe what happened during the session:

____

____

2. What did you learn in this session?

____

____

3. How do you think what you learnt in this session will be useful for you?

____

____

____

____

Signature of the Teacher Domain: K/A/S/C Level Attained: K/KH/SH/P

Session: 5

Name(s) of the faculty: ____________________

Date: ____________________ Time: ____________ to ____________

Duration: ____________________

Learning objective(s) of the session (Write from the presentation or as instructed by the faculty):

1. ____________________
2. ____________________
3. ____________________
4. ____________________

Teaching learning method(s) used in this session: ____________________

Reflections

1. Please describe what happened during the session:

____

____

2. What did you learn in this session?

____

____

3. How do you think what you learnt in this session will be useful for you?

____

____

____

____

Signature of the Teacher Domain: K/A/S/C Level Attained: K/KH/SH/P

Session: 6

Name(s) of the faculty: ____________________

Date: ____________________ Time: ____________ to ____________

Duration: ____________________

Learning objective(s) of the session (Write from the presentation or as instructed by the faculty):

1. ____________________
2. ____________________
3. ____________________
4. ____________________

Teaching learning method(s) used in this session: ____________________

Reflections

1. Please describe what happened during the session:

____

____

2. What did you learn in this session?

____

____

3. How do you think what you learnt in this session will be useful for you?

____

____

____

____

Signature of the Teacher Domain: K/A/S/C Level Attained: K/KH/SH/P

Session: 7

Name(s) of the faculty: ____________________

Date: ____________________ Time: __________ to __________

Duration: ____________________

Learning objective(s) of the session (Write from the presentation or as instructed by the faculty):

1. ____________________
2. ____________________
3. ____________________
4. ____________________

Teaching learning method(s) used in this session: ____________________

Reflections

1. Please describe what happened during the session:

____

____

2. What did you learn in this session?

____

____

3. How do you think what you learnt in this session will be useful for you?

____

____

____

____

Signature of the Teacher Domain: K/A/S/C Level Attained: K/KH/SH/P

Session: 8

Name(s) of the faculty: ____________________

Date: ____________________ Time: ____________ to ____________

Duration: ____________________

Learning objective(s) of the session (Write from the presentation or as instructed by the faculty):

1. ____________________
2. ____________________
3. ____________________
4. ____________________

Teaching learning method(s) used in this session: ____________________

Reflections

1. Please describe what happened during the session:

____

____

2. What did you learn in this session?

____

____

3. How do you think what you learnt in this session will be useful for you?

____

____

____

____

Signature of the Teacher Domain: K/A/S/C Level Attained: K/KH/SH/P

Session: 9

Name(s) of the faculty: ____________________

Date: ____________________ Time: ____________ to ____________

Duration: ____________________

Learning objective(s) of the session (Write from the presentation or as instructed by the faculty):

1. ____________________
2. ____________________
3. ____________________
4. ____________________

Teaching learning method(s) used in this session: ____________________

Reflections

1. Please describe what happened during the session:

____

____

2. What did you learn in this session?

____

____

3. How do you think what you learnt in this session will be useful for you?

____

____

____

____

Signature of the Teacher Domain: K/A/S/C Level Attained: K/KH/SH/P

Session: 10

Name(s) of the faculty: ____________________

Date: ____________________ Time: ____________ to ____________

Duration: ____________________

Learning objective(s) of the session (Write from the presentation or as instructed by the faculty):

1. ____________________
2. ____________________
3. ____________________
4. ____________________

Teaching learning method(s) used in this session: ____________________

Reflections

1. Please describe what happened during the session:

____

____

2. What did you learn in this session?

____

____

3. How do you think what you learnt in this session will be useful for you?

____

____

____

____

Signature of the Teacher Domain: K/A/S/C Level Attained: K/KH/SH/P

Session: 11

Name(s) of the faculty: ____________________

Date: ____________________ Time: ____________ to ____________

Duration: ____________________

Learning objective(s) of the session (Write from the presentation or as instructed by the faculty):

1. ____________________
2. ____________________
3. ____________________
4. ____________________

Teaching learning method(s) used in this session: ____________________

Reflections

1. Please describe what happened during the session:

____

____

2. What did you learn in this session?

____

____

3. How do you think what you learnt in this session will be useful for you?

____

____

____

____

Signature of the Teacher Domain: K/A/S/C Level Attained: K/KH/SH/P

Session: 12

Name(s) of the faculty: ____________________

Date: ____________________ Time: ____________ to ____________

Duration: ____________________

Learning objective(s) of the session (Write from the presentation or as instructed by the faculty):

1. ____________________
2. ____________________
3. ____________________
4. ____________________

Teaching learning method(s) used in this session: ____________________

Reflections

1. Please describe what happened during the session:

____

____

2. What did you learn in this session?

____

____

3. How do you think what you learnt in this session will be useful for you?

____

____

____

____

Signature of the Teacher Domain: K/A/S/C Level Attained: K/KH/SH/P

Session: 13

Name(s) of the faculty: ____________________

Date: ____________________ Time: ____________ to ____________

Duration: ____________________

Learning objective(s) of the session (Write from the presentation or as instructed by the faculty):

1. ____________________
2. ____________________
3. ____________________
4. ____________________

Teaching learning method(s) used in this session: ____________________

Reflections

1. Please describe what happened during the session:

____

____

2. What did you learn in this session?

____

____

3. How do you think what you learnt in this session will be useful for you?

____

____

____

____

Signature of the Teacher Domain: K/A/S/C Level Attained: K/KH/SH/P

Session: 14

Name(s) of the faculty: ____________________

Date: ____________________ Time: ____________ to ____________

Duration: ____________________

Learning objective(s) of the session (Write from the presentation or as instructed by the faculty):

1. ____________________
2. ____________________
3. ____________________
4. ____________________

Teaching learning method(s) used in this session: ____________________

Reflections

1. Please describe what happened during the session:

____

____

2. What did you learn in this session?

____

____

3. How do you think what you learnt in this session will be useful for you?

____

____

____

____

Signature of the Teacher Domain: K/A/S/C Level Attained: K/KH/SH/P

Session: 15

Name(s) of the faculty: ____________________

Date: ____________________ Time: ____________ to ____________

Duration: ____________________

Learning objective(s) of the session (Write from the presentation or as instructed by the faculty):

1. ____________________
2. ____________________
3. ____________________
4. ____________________

Teaching learning method(s) used in this session: ____________________

Reflections

1. Please describe what happened during the session:

____

____

2. What did you learn in this session?

____

____

3. How do you think what you learnt in this session will be useful for you?

____

____

____

____

Signature of the Teacher Domain: K/A/S/C Level Attained: K/KH/SH/P

Professional Development and Ethics Module

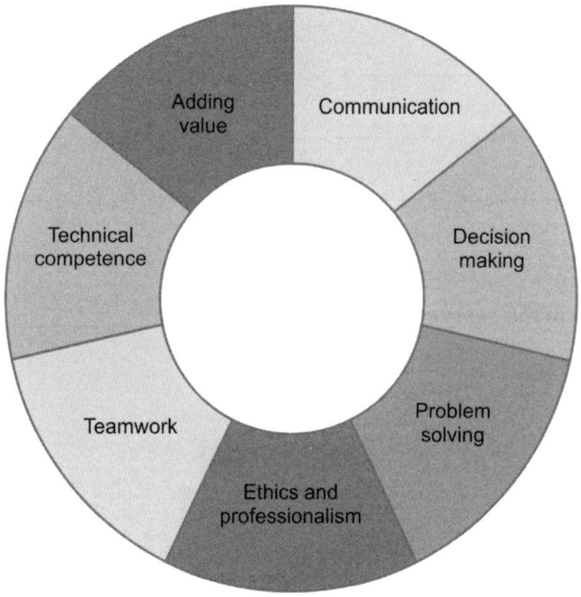

Session: 1

Name(s) of the faculty: ______________________________

Date: ____________________ Time: ____________ to ____________

Duration: ____________________

Learning objective(s) of the session (Write from the presentation or as instructed by the faculty):

1. ______________________________
2. ______________________________
3. ______________________________
4. ______________________________

Teaching learning method(s) used in this session: ______________________________

Reflections

1. Please describe what happened during the session:

____

____

2. What did you learn in this session?

____

____

3. How do you think what you learnt in this session will be useful for you?

____

____

____

____

Signature of the Teacher Domain: K/A/S/C Level Attained: K/KH/SH/P

Session: 2

Name(s) of the faculty: ______________________________

Date: ____________________ Time: ____________ to ____________

Duration: ____________________

Learning objective(s) of the session (Write from the presentation or as instructed by the faculty):

1. ______________________________
2. ______________________________
3. ______________________________
4. ______________________________

Teaching learning method(s) used in this session: ______________________________

Reflections

1. Please describe what happened during the session:

____

____

2. What did you learn in this session?

____

____

3. How do you think what you learnt in this session will be useful for you?

____

____

____

____

Signature of the Teacher Domain: K/A/S/C Level Attained: K/KH/SH/P

Session: 3

Name(s) of the faculty: ______________________________

Date: ____________________ Time: ____________ to ____________

Duration: ____________________

Learning objective(s) of the session (Write from the presentation or as instructed by the faculty):

1. ______________________________
2. ______________________________
3. ______________________________
4. ______________________________

Teaching learning method(s) used in this session: ______________________________

Reflections

1. Please describe what happened during the session:

____

____

2. What did you learn in this session?

____

____

3. How do you think what you learnt in this session will be useful for you?

____

____

____

____

Signature of the Teacher Domain: K/A/S/C Level Attained: K/KH/SH/P

Session: 4

Name(s) of the faculty: ____________________

Date: ____________________ Time: ____________ to ____________

Duration: ____________________

Learning objective(s) of the session (Write from the presentation or as instructed by the faculty):

1. ____________________
2. ____________________
3. ____________________
4. ____________________

Teaching learning method(s) used in this session: ____________________

Reflections

1. Please describe what happened during the session:

____

____

2. What did you learn in this session?

____

____

3. How do you think what you learnt in this session will be useful for you?

____

____

____

____

Signature of the Teacher Domain: K/A/S/C Level Attained: K/KH/SH/P

Session: 5

Name(s) of the faculty: ______________________________

Date: ____________________ Time: ____________ to ____________

Duration: ____________________

Learning objective(s) of the session (Write from the presentation or as instructed by the faculty):

1. ______________________________
2. ______________________________
3. ______________________________
4. ______________________________

Teaching learning method(s) used in this session: ______________________________

Reflections

1. Please describe what happened during the session:

____

____

2. What did you learn in this session?

____

____

3. How do you think what you learnt in this session will be useful for you?

____

____

____

____

Signature of the Teacher Domain: K/A/S/C Level Attained: K/KH/SH/P

Session: 6

Name(s) of the faculty: ____________________

Date: ____________________ Time: ____________ to ____________

Duration: ____________________

Learning objective(s) of the session (Write from the presentation or as instructed by the faculty):

1. ____________________
2. ____________________
3. ____________________
4. ____________________

Teaching learning method(s) used in this session: ____________________

Reflections

1. Please describe what happened during the session:

____

____

2. What did you learn in this session?

____

____

3. How do you think what you learnt in this session will be useful for you?

____

____

____

____

Signature of the Teacher Domain: K/A/S/C Level Attained: K/KH/SH/P

Session: 7

Name(s) of the faculty: ______________________________

Date: ____________________ Time: ____________ to ____________

Duration: ____________________

Learning objective(s) of the session (Write from the presentation or as instructed by the faculty):

1. ______________________________
2. ______________________________
3. ______________________________
4. ______________________________

Teaching learning method(s) used in this session: ______________________________

Reflections

1. Please describe what happened during the session:

____

____

2. What did you learn in this session?

____

____

3. How do you think what you learnt in this session will be useful for you?

____

____

____

____

Signature of the Teacher Domain: K/A/S/C Level Attained: K/KH/SH/P

Session: 8

Name(s) of the faculty: ____________________

Date: ____________________ Time: ____________ to ____________

Duration: ____________________

Learning objective(s) of the session (Write from the presentation or as instructed by the faculty):

1. ____________________
2. ____________________
3. ____________________
4. ____________________

Teaching learning method(s) used in this session: ____________________

Reflections

1. Please describe what happened during the session:

____

____

2. What did you learn in this session?

____

____

3. How do you think what you learnt in this session will be useful for you?

____

____

____

____

Signature of the Teacher Domain: K/A/S/C Level Attained: K/KH/SH/P

Session: 9

Name(s) of the faculty: ____________________

Date: ____________________ Time: ____________ to ____________

Duration: ____________________

Learning objective(s) of the session (Write from the presentation or as instructed by the faculty):

1. ____________________
2. ____________________
3. ____________________
4. ____________________

Teaching learning method(s) used in this session: ____________________

Reflections

1. Please describe what happened during the session:

____

____

2. What did you learn in this session?

____

____

3. How do you think what you learnt in this session will be useful for you?

____

____

____

____

Signature of the Teacher Domain: K/A/S/C Level Attained: K/KH/SH/P

Session: 10

Name(s) of the faculty: ______________________________

Date: ____________________ Time: ______________ to ______________

Duration: ____________________

Learning objective(s) of the session (Write from the presentation or as instructed by the faculty):

1. ______________________________
2. ______________________________
3. ______________________________
4. ______________________________

Teaching learning method(s) used in this session: ______________________________

Reflections

1. Please describe what happened during the session:

____

____

2. What did you learn in this session?

____

____

3. How do you think what you learnt in this session will be useful for you?

____

____

____

____

Signature of the Teacher Domain: K/A/S/C Level Attained: K/KH/SH/P

Session: 11

Name(s) of the faculty: ________________________________

Date: ____________________ Time: ____________ to ____________

Duration: ____________________

Learning objective(s) of the session (Write from the presentation or as instructed by the faculty):

1. ________________________________
2. ________________________________
3. ________________________________
4. ________________________________

Teaching learning method(s) used in this session: ________________________________

Reflections

1. Please describe what happened during the session:

____

____

2. What did you learn in this session?

____

____

3. How do you think what you learnt in this session will be useful for you?

____

____

____

____

Signature of the Teacher Domain: K/A/S/C Level Attained: K/KH/SH/P

Session: 12

Name(s) of the faculty: ____________________

Date: ____________________ Time: ____________ to ____________

Duration: ____________________

Learning objective(s) of the session (Write from the presentation or as instructed by the faculty):

1. ____________________
2. ____________________
3. ____________________
4. ____________________

Teaching learning method(s) used in this session: ____________________

Reflections

1. Please describe what happened during the session:

____

____

2. What did you learn in this session?

____

____

3. How do you think what you learnt in this session will be useful for you?

____

____

____

____

Signature of the Teacher Domain: K/A/S/C Level Attained: K/KH/SH/P

Session: 13

Name(s) of the faculty: ____________________

Date: ____________________ Time: ____________ to ____________

Duration: ____________________

Learning objective(s) of the session (Write from the presentation or as instructed by the faculty):

1. ____________________
2. ____________________
3. ____________________
4. ____________________

Teaching learning method(s) used in this session: ____________________

Reflections

1. Please describe what happened during the session:

____

____

2. What did you learn in this session?

____

____

3. How do you think what you learnt in this session will be useful for you?

____

____

____

____

Signature of the Teacher Domain: K/A/S/C Level Attained: K/KH/SH/P

Session: 14

Name(s) of the faculty: ______________________________

Date: ____________________ Time: ______________ to ______________

Duration: ____________________

Learning objective(s) of the session (Write from the presentation or as instructed by the faculty):

1. ______________________________
2. ______________________________
3. ______________________________
4. ______________________________

Teaching learning method(s) used in this session: ______________________________

Reflections

1. Please describe what happened during the session:

____

____

2. What did you learn in this session?

____

____

3. How do you think what you learnt in this session will be useful for you?

____

____

____

____

Signature of the Teacher Domain: K/A/S/C Level Attained: K/KH/SH/P

Session: 15

Name(s) of the faculty: ______________________________

Date: ____________________ Time: ______________ to ______________

Duration: ____________________

Learning objective(s) of the session (Write from the presentation or as instructed by the faculty):

1. ______________________________
2. ______________________________
3. ______________________________
4. ______________________________

Teaching learning method(s) used in this session: ______________________________

Reflections

1. Please describe what happened during the session:

____

____

2. What did you learn in this session?

____

____

3. How do you think what you learnt in this session will be useful for you?

____

____

____

____

Signature of the Teacher Domain: K/A/S/C Level Attained: K/KH/SH/P

Session: 16

Name(s) of the faculty: ____________________

Date: ____________________ Time: ____________ to ____________

Duration: ____________________

Learning objective(s) of the session (Write from the presentation or as instructed by the faculty):

1. ____________________
2. ____________________
3. ____________________
4. ____________________

Teaching learning method(s) used in this session: ____________________

Reflections

1. Please describe what happened during the session:

____

____

2. What did you learn in this session?

____

____

3. How do you think what you learnt in this session will be useful for you?

____

____

____

____

Signature of the Teacher Domain: K/A/S/C Level Attained: K/KH/SH/P

Session: 17

Name(s) of the faculty: ____________________

Date: ____________________ Time: ____________ to ____________

Duration: ____________________

Learning objective(s) of the session (Write from the presentation or as instructed by the faculty):

1. ____________________
2. ____________________
3. ____________________
4. ____________________

Teaching learning method(s) used in this session: ____________________

Reflections

1. Please describe what happened during the session:

____

____

2. What did you learn in this session?

____

____

3. How do you think what you learnt in this session will be useful for you?

____

____

____

____

Signature of the Teacher Domain: K/A/S/C Level Attained: K/KH/SH/P

Session: 18

Name(s) of the faculty: ____________________

Date: ____________________ Time: ____________ to ____________

Duration: ____________________

Learning objective(s) of the session (Write from the presentation or as instructed by the faculty):

1. ____________________
2. ____________________
3. ____________________
4. ____________________

Teaching learning method(s) used in this session: ____________________

Reflections

1. Please describe what happened during the session:

____

____

2. What did you learn in this session?

____

____

3. How do you think what you learnt in this session will be useful for you?

____

____

____

____

Signature of the Teacher Domain: K/A/S/C Level Attained: K/KH/SH/P

Session: 19

Name(s) of the faculty: ____________________

Date: ____________________ Time: ____________ to ____________

Duration: ____________________

Learning objective(s) of the session (Write from the presentation or as instructed by the faculty):

1. ____________________
2. ____________________
3. ____________________
4. ____________________

Teaching learning method(s) used in this session: ____________________

Reflections

1. Please describe what happened during the session:

____

____

2. What did you learn in this session?

____

____

3. How do you think what you learnt in this session will be useful for you?

____

____

____

____

Signature of the Teacher Domain: K/A/S/C Level Attained: K/KH/SH/P

Session: 20

Name(s) of the faculty: ____________________

Date: ____________________ Time: ____________ to ____________

Duration: ____________________

Learning objective(s) of the session (Write from the presentation or as instructed by the faculty):

1. ____________________
2. ____________________
3. ____________________
4. ____________________

Teaching learning method(s) used in this session: ____________________

Reflections

1. Please describe what happened during the session:

____

____

2. What did you learn in this session?

____

____

3. How do you think what you learnt in this session will be useful for you?

____

____

____

____

Signature of the Teacher Domain: K/A/S/C Level Attained: K/KH/SH/P

Session: 21

Name(s) of the faculty: ____________________

Date: ____________________ Time: ____________ to ____________

Duration: ____________________

Learning objective(s) of the session (Write from the presentation or as instructed by the faculty):

1. ____________________
2. ____________________
3. ____________________
4. ____________________

Teaching learning method(s) used in this session: ____________________

Reflections

1. Please describe what happened during the session:

____

____

2. What did you learn in this session?

____

____

3. How do you think what you learnt in this session will be useful for you?

____

____

____

____

Signature of the Teacher Domain: K/A/S/C Level Attained: K/KH/SH/P

Session: 22

Name(s) of the faculty: ______________________________

Date: ____________________ Time: ______________ to ______________

Duration: ____________________

Learning objective(s) of the session (Write from the presentation or as instructed by the faculty):

1. ______________________________
2. ______________________________
3. ______________________________
4. ______________________________

Teaching learning method(s) used in this session: ______________________________

Reflections

1. Please describe what happened during the session:

____

____

2. What did you learn in this session?

____

____

3. How do you think what you learnt in this session will be useful for you?

____

____

____

____

Signature of the Teacher Domain: K/A/S/C Level Attained: K/KH/SH/P

Session: 23

Name(s) of the faculty: ____________________

Date: ____________________ Time: ____________ to ____________

Duration: ____________________

Learning objective(s) of the session (Write from the presentation or as instructed by the faculty):

1. ____________________
2. ____________________
3. ____________________
4. ____________________

Teaching learning method(s) used in this session: ____________________

Reflections

1. Please describe what happened during the session:

____

____

2. What did you learn in this session?

____

____

3. How do you think what you learnt in this session will be useful for you?

____

____

____

____

Signature of the Teacher Domain: K/A/S/C Level Attained: K/KH/SH/P

Session: 24

Name(s) of the faculty: ______________________________

Date: ____________________ Time: ____________ to ____________

Duration: ____________________

Learning objective(s) of the session (Write from the presentation or as instructed by the faculty):

1. ______________________________
2. ______________________________
3. ______________________________
4. ______________________________

Teaching learning method(s) used in this session: ______________________________

Reflections

1. Please describe what happened during the session:

____

____

2. What did you learn in this session?

____

____

3. How do you think what you learnt in this session will be useful for you?

____

____

____

____

Signature of the Teacher Domain: K/A/S/C Level Attained: K/KH/SH/P

Session: 25

Name(s) of the faculty: ____________________

Date: ____________________ Time: ____________ to ____________

Duration: ____________________

Learning objective(s) of the session (Write from the presentation or as instructed by the faculty):

1. ____________________
2. ____________________
3. ____________________
4. ____________________

Teaching learning method(s) used in this session: ____________________

Reflections

1. Please describe what happened during the session:

____

____

2. What did you learn in this session?

____

____

3. How do you think what you learnt in this session will be useful for you?

____

____

____

____

Signature of the Teacher Domain: K/A/S/C Level Attained: K/KH/SH/P

Session: 26

Name(s) of the faculty: ____________________

Date: ____________________ Time: ____________ to ____________

Duration: ____________________

Learning objective(s) of the session (Write from the presentation or as instructed by the faculty):

1. ____________________
2. ____________________
3. ____________________
4. ____________________

Teaching learning method(s) used in this session: ____________________

Reflections

1. Please describe what happened during the session:

____

____

2. What did you learn in this session?

____

____

3. How do you think what you learnt in this session will be useful for you?

____

____

____

____

Signature of the Teacher Domain: K/A/S/C Level Attained: K/KH/SH/P

Session: 27

Name(s) of the faculty: ______________________________

Date: ____________________ Time: ______________ to ______________

Duration: ____________________

Learning objective(s) of the session (Write from the presentation or as instructed by the faculty):

1. ______________________________
2. ______________________________
3. ______________________________
4. ______________________________

Teaching learning method(s) used in this session: ______________________________

Reflections

1. Please describe what happened during the session:

____

____

2. What did you learn in this session?

____

____

3. How do you think what you learnt in this session will be useful for you?

____

____

____

____

Signature of the Teacher Domain: K/A/S/C Level Attained: K/KH/SH/P

Session: 28

Name(s) of the faculty: ____________________

Date: ____________________ Time: __________ to __________

Duration: ____________________

Learning objective(s) of the session (Write from the presentation or as instructed by the faculty):

1. ____________________
2. ____________________
3. ____________________
4. ____________________

Teaching learning method(s) used in this session: ____________________

Reflections

1. Please describe what happened during the session:

____

____

2. What did you learn in this session?

____

____

3. How do you think what you learnt in this session will be useful for you?

____

____

____

____

Signature of the Teacher Domain: K/A/S/C Level Attained: K/KH/SH/P

Session: 29

Name(s) of the faculty: ____________________

Date: ____________________ Time: ____________ to ____________

Duration: ____________________

Learning objective(s) of the session (Write from the presentation or as instructed by the faculty):

1. ____________________
2. ____________________
3. ____________________
4. ____________________

Teaching learning method(s) used in this session: ____________________

Reflections

1. Please describe what happened during the session:

____

____

2. What did you learn in this session?

____

____

3. How do you think what you learnt in this session will be useful for you?

____

____

____

____

Signature of the Teacher Domain: K/A/S/C Level Attained: K/KH/SH/P

Session: 30

Name(s) of the faculty: ____________________

Date: ____________________ Time: ____________ to ____________

Duration: ____________________

Learning objective(s) of the session (Write from the presentation or as instructed by the faculty):

1. ____________________
2. ____________________
3. ____________________
4. ____________________

Teaching learning method(s) used in this session: ____________________

Reflections

1. Please describe what happened during the session:

____

____

2. What did you learn in this session?

____

____

3. How do you think what you learnt in this session will be useful for you?

____

____

____

____

Signature of the Teacher Domain: K/A/S/C Level Attained: K/KH/SH/P

Session: 31

Name(s) of the faculty: ______

Date: ______ Time: ______ to ______

Duration: ______

Learning objective(s) of the session (Write from the presentation or as instructed by the faculty):

1. ______
2. ______
3. ______
4. ______

Teaching learning method(s) used in this session: ______

Reflections

1. Please describe what happened during the session:

______

______

2. What did you learn in this session?

______

______

3. How do you think what you learnt in this session will be useful for you?

______

______

______

______

Signature of the Teacher Domain: K/A/S/C Level Attained: K/KH/SH/P

Session: 32

Name(s) of the faculty: ______________________________

Date: ______________________ Time: ______________ to ______________

Duration: ______________________

Learning objective(s) of the session (Write from the presentation or as instructed by the faculty):

1. ______________________________
2. ______________________________
3. ______________________________
4. ______________________________

Teaching learning method(s) used in this session: ______________________________

Reflections

1. Please describe what happened during the session:

____

____

2. What did you learn in this session?

____

____

3. How do you think what you learnt in this session will be useful for you?

____

____

____

____

Signature of the Teacher Domain: K/A/S/C Level Attained: K/KH/SH/P

Session: 33

Name(s) of the faculty: ____________________

Date: ____________________ Time: ____________ to ____________

Duration: ____________________

Learning objective(s) of the session (Write from the presentation or as instructed by the faculty):

1. ____________________
2. ____________________
3. ____________________
4. ____________________

Teaching learning method(s) used in this session: ____________________

Reflections

1. Please describe what happened during the session:

____

____

2. What did you learn in this session?

____

____

3. How do you think what you learnt in this session will be useful for you?

____

____

____

____

Signature of the Teacher Domain: K/A/S/C Level Attained: K/KH/SH/P

Session: 34

Name(s) of the faculty: ____________________

Date: ____________________ Time: ____________ to ____________

Duration: ____________________

Learning objective(s) of the session (Write from the presentation or as instructed by the faculty):

1. ____________________
2. ____________________
3. ____________________
4. ____________________

Teaching learning method(s) used in this session: ____________________

Reflections

1. Please describe what happened during the session:

____

____

2. What did you learn in this session?

____

____

3. How do you think what you learnt in this session will be useful for you?

____

____

____

____

Signature of the Teacher Domain: K/A/S/C Level Attained: K/KH/SH/P

Session: 35

Name(s) of the faculty: ____________________

Date: ____________________ Time: ____________ to ____________

Duration: ____________________

Learning objective(s) of the session (Write from the presentation or as instructed by the faculty):

1. ____________________
2. ____________________
3. ____________________
4. ____________________

Teaching learning method(s) used in this session: ____________________

Reflections

1. Please describe what happened during the session:

____

____

2. What did you learn in this session?

____

____

3. How do you think what you learnt in this session will be useful for you?

____

____

____

____

Signature of the Teacher Domain: K/A/S/C Level Attained: K/KH/SH/P

Session: 36

Name(s) of the faculty: ____________________

Date: ____________________ Time: ____________ to ____________

Duration: ____________________

Learning objective(s) of the session (Write from the presentation or as instructed by the faculty):

1. ____________________
2. ____________________
3. ____________________
4. ____________________

Teaching learning method(s) used in this session: ____________________

Reflections

1. Please describe what happened during the session:

____

____

2. What did you learn in this session?

____

____

3. How do you think what you learnt in this session will be useful for you?

____

____

____

____

Signature of the Teacher Domain: K/A/S/C Level Attained: K/KH/SH/P

Session: 37

Name(s) of the faculty: ______________________________

Date: ____________________ Time: ______________ to ______________

Duration: ____________________

Learning objective(s) of the session (Write from the presentation or as instructed by the faculty):

1. ______________________________
2. ______________________________
3. ______________________________
4. ______________________________

Teaching learning method(s) used in this session: ______________________________

Reflections

1. Please describe what happened during the session:

____

____

2. What did you learn in this session?

____

____

3. How do you think what you learnt in this session will be useful for you?

____

____

____

____

Signature of the Teacher Domain: K/A/S/C Level Attained: K/KH/SH/P

Session: 38

Name(s) of the faculty: ____________________

Date: ____________________ Time: ____________ to ____________

Duration: ____________________

Learning objective(s) of the session (Write from the presentation or as instructed by the faculty):

1. ____________________
2. ____________________
3. ____________________
4. ____________________

Teaching learning method(s) used in this session: ____________________

Reflections

1. Please describe what happened during the session:

____

____

2. What did you learn in this session?

____

____

3. How do you think what you learnt in this session will be useful for you?

____

____

____

____

Signature of the Teacher Domain: K/A/S/C Level Attained: K/KH/SH/P

Session: 39

Name(s) of the faculty: ____________________

Date: ____________________ Time: ____________ to ____________

Duration: ____________________

Learning objective(s) of the session (Write from the presentation or as instructed by the faculty):

1. ____________________
2. ____________________
3. ____________________
4. ____________________

Teaching learning method(s) used in this session: ____________________

Reflections

1. Please describe what happened during the session:

____

____

2. What did you learn in this session?

____

____

3. How do you think what you learnt in this session will be useful for you?

____

____

____

____

Signature of the Teacher Domain: K/A/S/C Level Attained: K/KH/SH/P

Session: 40

Name(s) of the faculty: ____________________

Date: ____________________ Time: ____________ to ____________

Duration: ____________________

Learning objective(s) of the session (Write from the presentation or as instructed by the faculty):

1. ____________________
2. ____________________
3. ____________________
4. ____________________

Teaching learning method(s) used in this session: ____________________

Reflections

1. Please describe what happened during the session:

____

____

2. What did you learn in this session?

____

____

3. How do you think what you learnt in this session will be useful for you?

____

____

____

____

Signature of the Teacher Domain: K/A/S/C Level Attained: K/KH/SH/P

Enhancement of Language and Computer Skills Module

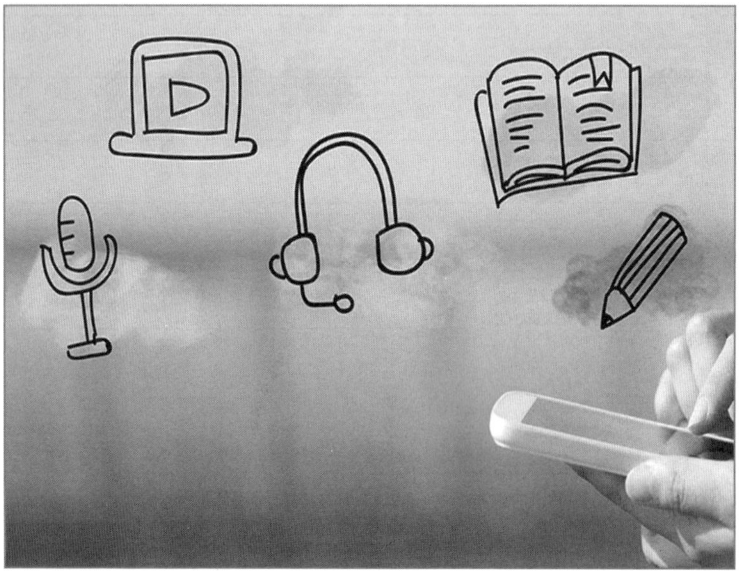

Session: 1

Name(s) of the faculty: ____________________

Date: ____________________ Time: ____________ to ____________

Duration: ____________________

Learning objective(s) of the session (Write from the presentation or as instructed by the faculty):

1. ____________________
2. ____________________
3. ____________________
4. ____________________

Teaching learning method(s) used in this session: ____________________

Reflections

1. Please describe what happened during the session:

____

____

2. What did you learn in this session?

____

____

3. How do you think what you learnt in this session will be useful for you?

____

____

____

____

Signature of the Teacher Domain: K/A/S/C Level Attained: K/KH/SH/P

Session: 2

Name(s) of the faculty: ____________________

Date: ____________________ Time: ____________ to ____________

Duration: ____________________

Learning objective(s) of the session (Write from the presentation or as instructed by the faculty):

1. ____________________
2. ____________________
3. ____________________
4. ____________________

Teaching learning method(s) used in this session: ____________________

Reflections

1. Please describe what happened during the session:

____

____

2. What did you learn in this session?

____

____

3. How do you think what you learnt in this session will be useful for you?

____

____

____

____

Signature of the Teacher Domain: K/A/S/C Level Attained: K/KH/SH/P

Session: 3

Name(s) of the faculty: ______________________________

Date: ____________________ Time: ______________ to ______________

Duration: ____________________

Learning objective(s) of the session (Write from the presentation or as instructed by the faculty):

1. ______________________________
2. ______________________________
3. ______________________________
4. ______________________________

Teaching learning method(s) used in this session: ______________________________

Reflections

1. Please describe what happened during the session:

____

____

2. What did you learn in this session?

____

____

3. How do you think what you learnt in this session will be useful for you?

____

____

____

____

Signature of the Teacher Domain: K/A/S/C Level Attained: K/KH/SH/P

Session: 4

Name(s) of the faculty: ____________________

Date: ____________________ Time: ____________ to ____________

Duration: ____________________

Learning objective(s) of the session (Write from the presentation or as instructed by the faculty):

1. ____________________
2. ____________________
3. ____________________
4. ____________________

Teaching learning method(s) used in this session: ____________________

Reflections

1. Please describe what happened during the session:

____

____

2. What did you learn in this session?

____

____

3. How do you think what you learnt in this session will be useful for you?

____

____

____

____

Signature of the Teacher Domain: K/A/S/C Level Attained: K/KH/SH/P

Session: 5

Name(s) of the faculty: ______________________________

Date: ____________________ Time: ______________ to ______________

Duration: ____________________

Learning objective(s) of the session (Write from the presentation or as instructed by the faculty):

1. ______________________________
2. ______________________________
3. ______________________________
4. ______________________________

Teaching learning method(s) used in this session: ______________________________

Reflections

1. Please describe what happened during the session:

____

____

2. What did you learn in this session?

____

____

3. How do you think what you learnt in this session will be useful for you?

____

____

____

____

Signature of the Teacher Domain: K/A/S/C Level Attained: K/KH/SH/P

Session: 6

Name(s) of the faculty: ______________________________

Date: ____________________ Time: ____________ to ____________

Duration: ____________________

Learning objective(s) of the session (Write from the presentation or as instructed by the faculty):

1. ______________________________
2. ______________________________
3. ______________________________
4. ______________________________

Teaching learning method(s) used in this session: ______________________________

Reflections

1. Please describe what happened during the session:

____

____

2. What did you learn in this session?

____

____

3. How do you think what you learnt in this session will be useful for you?

____

____

____

____

Signature of the Teacher Domain: K/A/S/C Level Attained: K/KH/SH/P

Session: 7

Name(s) of the faculty: ____________________

Date: ____________________ Time: ____________ to ____________

Duration: ____________________

Learning objective(s) of the session (Write from the presentation or as instructed by the faculty):

1. ____________________
2. ____________________
3. ____________________
4. ____________________

Teaching learning method(s) used in this session: ____________________

Reflections

1. Please describe what happened during the session:

____

____

2. What did you learn in this session?

____

____

3. How do you think what you learnt in this session will be useful for you?

____

____

____

____

Signature of the Teacher Domain: K/A/S/C Level Attained: K/KH/SH/P

Session: 8

Name(s) of the faculty: ____________________

Date: ____________________ Time: ____________ to ____________

Duration: ____________________

Learning objective(s) of the session (Write from the presentation or as instructed by the faculty):

1. ____________________
2. ____________________
3. ____________________
4. ____________________

Teaching learning method(s) used in this session: ____________________

Reflections

1. Please describe what happened during the session:

____

____

2. What did you learn in this session?

____

____

3. How do you think what you learnt in this session will be useful for you?

____

____

____

____

Signature of the Teacher Domain: K/A/S/C Level Attained: K/KH/SH/P

Session: 9

Name(s) of the faculty: ______________________________

Date: ____________________ Time: ____________ to ____________

Duration: ____________________

Learning objective(s) of the session (Write from the presentation or as instructed by the faculty):

1. ______________________________
2. ______________________________
3. ______________________________
4. ______________________________

Teaching learning method(s) used in this session: ______________________________

Reflections

1. Please describe what happened during the session:

____

____

2. What did you learn in this session?

____

____

3. How do you think what you learnt in this session will be useful for you?

____

____

____

____

Signature of the Teacher   Domain: K/A/S/C   Level Attained: K/KH/SH/P

Session: 10

Name(s) of the faculty: ____________________

Date: ____________________ Time: ____________ to ____________

Duration: ____________________

Learning objective(s) of the session (Write from the presentation or as instructed by the faculty):

1. ____________________
2. ____________________
3. ____________________
4. ____________________

Teaching learning method(s) used in this session: ____________________

Reflections

1. Please describe what happened during the session:

____

____

2. What did you learn in this session?

____

____

3. How do you think what you learnt in this session will be useful for you?

____

____

____

____

Signature of the Teacher Domain: K/A/S/C Level Attained: K/KH/SH/P

Session: 11

Name(s) of the faculty: ____________________

Date: ____________________ Time: ____________ to ____________

Duration: ____________________

Learning objective(s) of the session (Write from the presentation or as instructed by the faculty):

1. ____________________
2. ____________________
3. ____________________
4. ____________________

Teaching learning method(s) used in this session: ____________________

Reflections

1. Please describe what happened during the session:

____

____

2. What did you learn in this session?

____

____

3. How do you think what you learnt in this session will be useful for you?

____

____

____

____

Signature of the Teacher Domain: K/A/S/C Level Attained: K/KH/SH/P

Session: 12

Name(s) of the faculty: ______________________________

Date: ____________________ Time: ______________ to ______________

Duration: ____________________

Learning objective(s) of the session (Write from the presentation or as instructed by the faculty):

1. ______________________________
2. ______________________________
3. ______________________________
4. ______________________________

Teaching learning method(s) used in this session: ______________________________

Reflections

1. Please describe what happened during the session:

____

____

2. What did you learn in this session?

____

____

3. How do you think what you learnt in this session will be useful for you?

____

____

____

____

Signature of the Teacher Domain: K/A/S/C Level Attained: K/KH/SH/P

Session: 13

Name(s) of the faculty: ____________________

Date: ____________________ Time: ____________ to ____________

Duration: ____________________

Learning objective(s) of the session (Write from the presentation or as instructed by the faculty):

1. ____________________
2. ____________________
3. ____________________
4. ____________________

Teaching learning method(s) used in this session: ____________________

Reflections

1. Please describe what happened during the session:

____

____

2. What did you learn in this session?

____

____

3. How do you think what you learnt in this session will be useful for you?

____

____

____

____

Signature of the Teacher Domain: K/A/S/C Level Attained: K/KH/SH/P

Session: 14

Name(s) of the faculty: ______________________________

Date: ____________________ Time: ____________ to ____________

Duration: ____________________

Learning objective(s) of the session (Write from the presentation or as instructed by the faculty):

1. ______________________________
2. ______________________________
3. ______________________________
4. ______________________________

Teaching learning method(s) used in this session: ______________________________

Reflections

1. Please describe what happened during the session:

____

____

2. What did you learn in this session?

____

____

3. How do you think what you learnt in this session will be useful for you?

____

____

____

____

Signature of the Teacher Domain: K/A/S/C Level Attained: K/KH/SH/P

Session: 15

Name(s) of the faculty: ______________________________

Date: ____________________ Time: ______________ to ______________

Duration: ____________________

Learning objective(s) of the session (Write from the presentation or as instructed by the faculty):

1. ______________________________
2. ______________________________
3. ______________________________
4. ______________________________

Teaching learning method(s) used in this session: ______________________________

Reflections

1. Please describe what happened during the session:

____

____

2. What did you learn in this session?

____

____

3. How do you think what you learnt in this session will be useful for you?

____

____

____

____

Signature of the Teacher Domain: K/A/S/C Level Attained: K/KH/SH/P

Session: 16

Name(s) of the faculty: ____________________

Date: ____________________ Time: ____________ to ____________

Duration: ____________________

Learning objective(s) of the session (Write from the presentation or as instructed by the faculty):

1. ____________________
2. ____________________
3. ____________________
4. ____________________

Teaching learning method(s) used in this session: ____________________

Reflections

1. Please describe what happened during the session:

____

____

2. What did you learn in this session?

____

____

3. How do you think what you learnt in this session will be useful for you?

____

____

____

____

Signature of the Teacher Domain: K/A/S/C Level Attained: K/KH/SH/P

Session: 17

Name(s) of the faculty: ______________________________

Date: ______________________ Time: ______________ to ______________

Duration: ______________________

Learning objective(s) of the session (Write from the presentation or as instructed by the faculty):

1. ______________________________
2. ______________________________
3. ______________________________
4. ______________________________

Teaching learning method(s) used in this session: ______________________________

Reflections

1. Please describe what happened during the session:

____

____

2. What did you learn in this session?

____

____

3. How do you think what you learnt in this session will be useful for you?

____

____

____

____

Signature of the Teacher Domain: K/A/S/C Level Attained: K/KH/SH/P

Session: 18

Name(s) of the faculty: ____________________

Date: ____________________ Time: ____________ to ____________

Duration: ____________________

Learning objective(s) of the session (Write from the presentation or as instructed by the faculty):

1. ____________________
2. ____________________
3. ____________________
4. ____________________

Teaching learning method(s) used in this session: ____________________

Reflections

1. Please describe what happened during the session:

____

____

2. What did you learn in this session?

____

____

3. How do you think what you learnt in this session will be useful for you?

____

____

____

____

Signature of the Teacher Domain: K/A/S/C Level Attained: K/KH/SH/P

Session: 19

Name(s) of the faculty: ______________________________

Date: ____________________ Time: ____________ to ____________

Duration: ____________________

Learning objective(s) of the session (Write from the presentation or as instructed by the faculty):

1. ______________________________
2. ______________________________
3. ______________________________
4. ______________________________

Teaching learning method(s) used in this session: ______________________________

Reflections

1. Please describe what happened during the session:

____

____

2. What did you learn in this session?

____

____

3. How do you think what you learnt in this session will be useful for you?

____

____

____

____

Signature of the Teacher Domain: K/A/S/C Level Attained: K/KH/SH/P

Session: 20

Name(s) of the faculty: ______________________________

Date: ______________________ Time: ______________ to ______________

Duration: ______________________

Learning objective(s) of the session (Write from the presentation or as instructed by the faculty):

1. ______________________________
2. ______________________________
3. ______________________________
4. ______________________________

Teaching learning method(s) used in this session: ______________________________

Reflections

1. Please describe what happened during the session:

____

____

2. What did you learn in this session?

____

____

3. How do you think what you learnt in this session will be useful for you?

____

____

____

____

Signature of the Teacher Domain: K/A/S/C Level Attained: K/KH/SH/P

Session: 21

Name(s) of the faculty: ____________________

Date: ____________________ Time: ____________ to ____________

Duration: ____________________

Learning objective(s) of the session (Write from the presentation or as instructed by the faculty):

1. ____________________
2. ____________________
3. ____________________
4. ____________________

Teaching learning method(s) used in this session: ____________________

Reflections

1. Please describe what happened during the session:

____

____

2. What did you learn in this session?

____

____

3. How do you think what you learnt in this session will be useful for you?

____

____

____

____

Signature of the Teacher Domain: K/A/S/C Level Attained: K/KH/SH/P

Session: 22

Name(s) of the faculty: ____________________

Date: ____________________ Time: ____________ to ____________

Duration: ____________________

Learning objective(s) of the session (Write from the presentation or as instructed by the faculty):

1. ____________________
2. ____________________
3. ____________________
4. ____________________

Teaching learning method(s) used in this session: ____________________

Reflections

1. Please describe what happened during the session:

____

____

2. What did you learn in this session?

____

____

3. How do you think what you learnt in this session will be useful for you?

____

____

____

____

Signature of the Teacher Domain: K/A/S/C Level Attained: K/KH/SH/P

Session: 23

Name(s) of the faculty: ______________________________

Date: ____________________ Time: ____________ to ____________

Duration: ____________________

Learning objective(s) of the session (Write from the presentation or as instructed by the faculty):

1. ______________________________
2. ______________________________
3. ______________________________
4. ______________________________

Teaching learning method(s) used in this session: ______________________________

Reflections

1. Please describe what happened during the session:

____

____

2. What did you learn in this session?

____

____

3. How do you think what you learnt in this session will be useful for you?

____

____

____

____

Signature of the Teacher Domain: K/A/S/C Level Attained: K/KH/SH/P

Session: 24

Name(s) of the faculty: ____________________

Date: ____________________ Time: ____________ to ____________

Duration: ____________________

Learning objective(s) of the session (Write from the presentation or as instructed by the faculty):

1. ____________________
2. ____________________
3. ____________________
4. ____________________

Teaching learning method(s) used in this session: ____________________

Reflections

1. Please describe what happened during the session:

____

____

2. What did you learn in this session?

____

____

3. How do you think what you learnt in this session will be useful for you?

____

____

____

____

Signature of the Teacher Domain: K/A/S/C Level Attained: K/KH/SH/P

Session: 25

Name(s) of the faculty: ______________________________

Date: ______________________ Time: ______________ to ______________

Duration: ______________________

Learning objective(s) of the session (Write from the presentation or as instructed by the faculty):

1. ______________________________
2. ______________________________
3. ______________________________
4. ______________________________

Teaching learning method(s) used in this session: ______________________________

Reflections

1. Please describe what happened during the session:

____

____

2. What did you learn in this session?

____

____

3. How do you think what you learnt in this session will be useful for you?

____

____

____

____

Signature of the Teacher Domain: K/A/S/C Level Attained: K/KH/SH/P

Session: 26

Name(s) of the faculty: ____________________

Date: ____________________ Time: ____________ to ____________

Duration: ____________________

Learning objective(s) of the session (Write from the presentation or as instructed by the faculty):

1. ____________________
2. ____________________
3. ____________________
4. ____________________

Teaching learning method(s) used in this session: ____________________

Reflections

1. Please describe what happened during the session:

____

____

2. What did you learn in this session?

____

____

3. How do you think what you learnt in this session will be useful for you?

____

____

____

____

Signature of the Teacher Domain: K/A/S/C Level Attained: K/KH/SH/P

Session: 27

Name(s) of the faculty: ____________________

Date: ____________________ Time: ____________ to ____________

Duration: ____________________

Learning objective(s) of the session (Write from the presentation or as instructed by the faculty):

1. ____________________
2. ____________________
3. ____________________
4. ____________________

Teaching learning method(s) used in this session: ____________________

Reflections

1. Please describe what happened during the session:

____

____

2. What did you learn in this session?

____

____

3. How do you think what you learnt in this session will be useful for you?

____

____

____

____

Signature of the Teacher Domain: K/A/S/C Level Attained: K/KH/SH/P

Session: 28

Name(s) of the faculty: ____________________

Date: ____________________ Time: ____________ to ____________

Duration: ____________________

Learning objective(s) of the session (Write from the presentation or as instructed by the faculty):

1. ____________________
2. ____________________
3. ____________________
4. ____________________

Teaching learning method(s) used in this session: ____________________

Reflections

1. Please describe what happened during the session:

____

____

2. What did you learn in this session?

____

____

3. How do you think what you learnt in this session will be useful for you?

____

____

____

____

Signature of the Teacher Domain: K/A/S/C Level Attained: K/KH/SH/P

Session: 29

Name(s) of the faculty: ______________________________

Date: ____________________ Time: ______________ to ______________

Duration: ____________________

Learning objective(s) of the session (Write from the presentation or as instructed by the faculty):

1. ______________________________
2. ______________________________
3. ______________________________
4. ______________________________

Teaching learning method(s) used in this session: ______________________________

Reflections

1. Please describe what happened during the session:

____

____

2. What did you learn in this session?

____

____

3. How do you think what you learnt in this session will be useful for you?

____

____

____

____

Signature of the Teacher Domain: K/A/S/C Level Attained: K/KH/SH/P

Session: 30

Name(s) of the faculty: ______________________________

Date: ____________________ Time: ______________ to ______________

Duration: ____________________

Learning objective(s) of the session (Write from the presentation or as instructed by the faculty):

1. ______________________________
2. ______________________________
3. ______________________________
4. ______________________________

Teaching learning method(s) used in this session: ______________________________

Reflections

1. Please describe what happened during the session:

____

____

2. What did you learn in this session?

____

____

3. How do you think what you learnt in this session will be useful for you?

____

____

____

____

Signature of the Teacher Domain: K/A/S/C Level Attained: K/KH/SH/P

Session: 31

Name(s) of the faculty: ______________________________

Date: ____________________ Time: ____________ to ____________

Duration: ____________________

Learning objective(s) of the session (Write from the presentation or as instructed by the faculty):

1. ______________________________
2. ______________________________
3. ______________________________
4. ______________________________

Teaching learning method(s) used in this session: ______________________________

Reflections

1. Please describe what happened during the session:

____

____

2. What did you learn in this session?

____

____

3. How do you think what you learnt in this session will be useful for you?

____

____

____

____

Signature of the Teacher Domain: K/A/S/C Level Attained: K/KH/SH/P

Session: 32

Name(s) of the faculty: ______________________________

Date: ____________________ Time: ______________ to ______________

Duration: ____________________

Learning objective(s) of the session (Write from the presentation or as instructed by the faculty):

1. ______________________________
2. ______________________________
3. ______________________________
4. ______________________________

Teaching learning method(s) used in this session: ______________________________

Reflections

1. Please describe what happened during the session:

____

____

2. What did you learn in this session?

____

____

3. How do you think what you learnt in this session will be useful for you?

____

____

____

____

Signature of the Teacher Domain: K/A/S/C Level Attained: K/KH/SH/P

Session: 33

Name(s) of the faculty: ____________________

Date: ____________________ Time: __________ to __________

Duration: ____________________

Learning objective(s) of the session (Write from the presentation or as instructed by the faculty):

1. ____________________
2. ____________________
3. ____________________
4. ____________________

Teaching learning method(s) used in this session: ____________________

Reflections

1. Please describe what happened during the session:

____

____

2. What did you learn in this session?

____

____

3. How do you think what you learnt in this session will be useful for you?

____

____

____

____

Signature of the Teacher Domain: K/A/S/C Level Attained: K/KH/SH/P

Session: 34

Name(s) of the faculty: ______________________________

Date: ____________________ Time: ______________ to ______________

Duration: ____________________

Learning objective(s) of the session (Write from the presentation or as instructed by the faculty):

1. ______________________________
2. ______________________________
3. ______________________________
4. ______________________________

Teaching learning method(s) used in this session: ______________________________

Reflections

1. Please describe what happened during the session:

____

____

2. What did you learn in this session?

____

____

3. How do you think what you learnt in this session will be useful for you?

____

____

____

____

Signature of the Teacher Domain: K/A/S/C Level Attained: K/KH/SH/P

Session: 35

Name(s) of the faculty: ____________________

Date: ____________________ Time: ____________ to ____________

Duration: ____________________

Learning objective(s) of the session (Write from the presentation or as instructed by the faculty):

1. ____________________
2. ____________________
3. ____________________
4. ____________________

Teaching learning method(s) used in this session: ____________________

Reflections

1. Please describe what happened during the session:

____

____

2. What did you learn in this session?

____

____

3. How do you think what you learnt in this session will be useful for you?

____

____

____

____

Signature of the Teacher Domain: K/A/S/C Level Attained: K/KH/SH/P

Session: 36

Name(s) of the faculty: ______________________________

Date: ____________________ Time: ____________ to ____________

Duration: ____________________

Learning objective(s) of the session (Write from the presentation or as instructed by the faculty):

1. ______________________________
2. ______________________________
3. ______________________________
4. ______________________________

Teaching learning method(s) used in this session: ______________________________

Reflections

1. Please describe what happened during the session:

____

____

2. What did you learn in this session?

____

____

3. How do you think what you learnt in this session will be useful for you?

____

____

____

____

Signature of the Teacher Domain: K/A/S/C Level Attained: K/KH/SH/P

Session: 37

Name(s) of the faculty: ____________________

Date: ____________________ Time: ____________ to ____________

Duration: ____________________

Learning objective(s) of the session (Write from the presentation or as instructed by the faculty):

1. ____________________

2. ____________________

3. ____________________

4. ____________________

Teaching learning method(s) used in this session: ____________________

Reflections

1. Please describe what happened during the session:

____

____

2. What did you learn in this session?

____

____

3. How do you think what you learnt in this session will be useful for you?

____

____

____

____

Signature of the Teacher Domain: K/A/S/C Level Attained: K/KH/SH/P

Session: 38

Name(s) of the faculty: ______________________________

Date: ____________________ Time: ____________ to ____________

Duration: ____________________

Learning objective(s) of the session (Write from the presentation or as instructed by the faculty):

1. ______________________________
2. ______________________________
3. ______________________________
4. ______________________________

Teaching learning method(s) used in this session: ______________________________

Reflections

1. Please describe what happened during the session:

____

____

2. What did you learn in this session?

____

____

3. How do you think what you learnt in this session will be useful for you?

____

____

____

____

Signature of the Teacher Domain: K/A/S/C Level Attained: K/KH/SH/P

Session: 39

Name(s) of the faculty: ______________________________

Date: ____________________ Time: ____________ to ____________

Duration: ____________________

Learning objective(s) of the session (Write from the presentation or as instructed by the faculty):

1. ______________________________
2. ______________________________
3. ______________________________
4. ______________________________

Teaching learning method(s) used in this session: ______________________________

Reflections

1. Please describe what happened during the session:

____

____

2. What did you learn in this session?

____

____

3. How do you think what you learnt in this session will be useful for you?

____

____

____

____

Signature of the Teacher Domain: K/A/S/C Level Attained: K/KH/SH/P

Session: 40

Name(s) of the faculty: ____________________

Date: ____________________ Time: ____________ to ____________

Duration: ____________________

Learning objective(s) of the session (Write from the presentation or as instructed by the faculty):

1. ____________________
2. ____________________
3. ____________________
4. ____________________

Teaching learning method(s) used in this session: ____________________

Reflections

1. Please describe what happened during the session:

____

____

2. What did you learn in this session?

____

____

3. How do you think what you learnt in this session will be useful for you?

____

____

____

____

Signature of the Teacher Domain: K/A/S/C Level Attained: K/KH/SH/P

Sports and Extra-curricular Activities Module

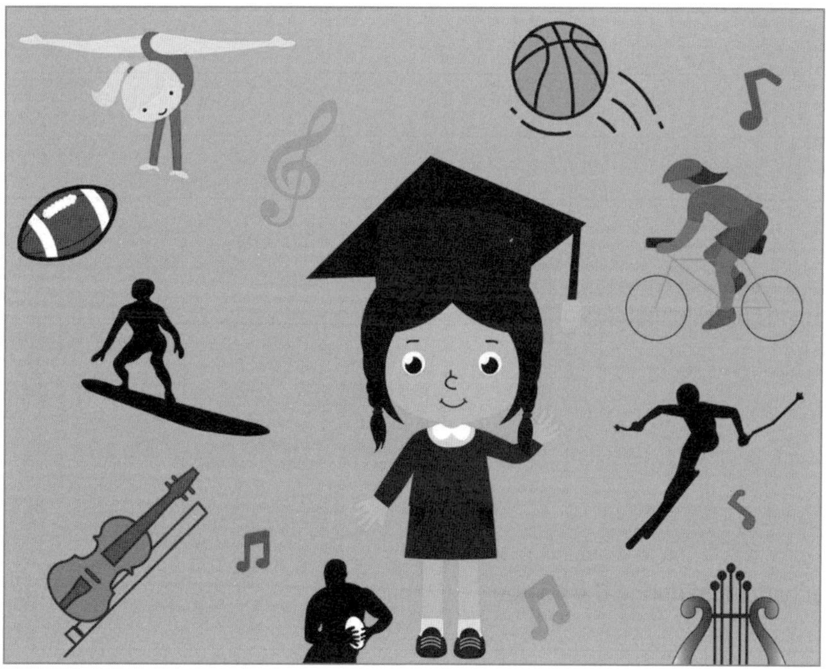

Session: 1

Name(s) of the faculty: ____________________

Date: ____________________ Time: ____________ to ____________

Duration: ____________________

Learning objective(s) of the session (Write from the presentation or as instructed by the faculty):

1. ____________________
2. ____________________
3. ____________________
4. ____________________

Teaching learning method(s) used in this session: ____________________

Reflections

1. Please describe what happened during the session:

____

____

2. What did you learn in this session?

____

____

3. How do you think what you learnt in this session will be useful for you?

____

____

____

____

Signature of the Teacher Domain: K/A/S/C Level Attained: K/KH/SH/P

Session: 2

Name(s) of the faculty: ____________________

Date: ____________________ Time: ______________ to ______________

Duration: ____________________

Learning objective(s) of the session (Write from the presentation or as instructed by the faculty):

1. ____________________
2. ____________________
3. ____________________
4. ____________________

Teaching learning method(s) used in this session: ____________________

Reflections

1. Please describe what happened during the session:

____

____

2. What did you learn in this session?

____

____

3. How do you think what you learnt in this session will be useful for you?

____

____

____

____

Signature of the Teacher Domain: K/A/S/C Level Attained: K/KH/SH/P

Session: 3

Name(s) of the faculty: ____________________

Date: ____________________ Time: __________ to __________

Duration: ____________________

Learning objective(s) of the session (Write from the presentation or as instructed by the faculty):

1. ____________________
2. ____________________
3. ____________________
4. ____________________

Teaching learning method(s) used in this session: ____________________

Reflections

1. Please describe what happened during the session:

____

____

2. What did you learn in this session?

____

____

3. How do you think what you learnt in this session will be useful for you?

____

____

____

____

Signature of the Teacher Domain: K/A/S/C Level Attained: K/KH/SH/P

Session: 4

Name(s) of the faculty: ____________________

Date: ____________________ Time: ____________ to ____________

Duration: ____________________

Learning objective(s) of the session (Write from the presentation or as instructed by the faculty):

1. ____________________
2. ____________________
3. ____________________
4. ____________________

Teaching learning method(s) used in this session: ____________________

Reflections

1. Please describe what happened during the session:

____

____

2. What did you learn in this session?

____

____

3. How do you think what you learnt in this session will be useful for you?

____

____

____

____

Signature of the Teacher Domain: K/A/S/C Level Attained: K/KH/SH/P

Session: 5

Name(s) of the faculty: ______________________________

Date: ____________________ Time: ____________ to ____________

Duration: ____________________

Learning objective(s) of the session (Write from the presentation or as instructed by the faculty):

1. ______________________________
2. ______________________________
3. ______________________________
4. ______________________________

Teaching learning method(s) used in this session: ______________________________

Reflections

1. Please describe what happened during the session:

____

____

2. What did you learn in this session?

____

____

3. How do you think what you learnt in this session will be useful for you?

____

____

____

____

Signature of the Teacher Domain: K/A/S/C Level Attained: K/KH/SH/P

Session: 6

Name(s) of the faculty: ______________________________

Date: ______________________ Time: ______________ to ______________

Duration: ______________________

Learning objective(s) of the session (Write from the presentation or as instructed by the faculty):

1. ______________________________
2. ______________________________
3. ______________________________
4. ______________________________

Teaching learning method(s) used in this session: ______________________________

Reflections

1. Please describe what happened during the session:

____

____

2. What did you learn in this session?

____

____

3. How do you think what you learnt in this session will be useful for you?

____

____

____

____

Signature of the Teacher Domain: K/A/S/C Level Attained: K/KH/SH/P

Session: 7

Name(s) of the faculty: ____________________

Date: ____________________ Time: ____________ to ____________

Duration: ____________________

Learning objective(s) of the session (Write from the presentation or as instructed by the faculty):

1. ____________________
2. ____________________
3. ____________________
4. ____________________

Teaching learning method(s) used in this session: ____________________

Reflections

1. Please describe what happened during the session:

____

____

2. What did you learn in this session?

____

____

3. How do you think what you learnt in this session will be useful for you?

____

____

____

____

Signature of the Teacher Domain: K/A/S/C Level Attained: K/KH/SH/P

Session: 8

Name(s) of the faculty: ______________________________

Date: ____________________ Time: ____________ to ____________

Duration: ____________________

Learning objective(s) of the session (Write from the presentation or as instructed by the faculty):

1. ______________________________
2. ______________________________
3. ______________________________
4. ______________________________

Teaching learning method(s) used in this session: ______________________________

Reflections

1. Please describe what happened during the session:

____

____

2. What did you learn in this session?

____

____

3. How do you think what you learnt in this session will be useful for you?

____

____

____

____

Signature of the Teacher Domain: K/A/S/C Level Attained: K/KH/SH/P

Session: 9

Name(s) of the faculty: ____________________

Date: ____________________ Time: __________ to __________

Duration: ____________________

Learning objective(s) of the session (Write from the presentation or as instructed by the faculty):

1. ____________________
2. ____________________
3. ____________________
4. ____________________

Teaching learning method(s) used in this session: ____________________

Reflections

1. Please describe what happened during the session:

____

____

2. What did you learn in this session?

____

____

3. How do you think what you learnt in this session will be useful for you?

____

____

____

____

Signature of the Teacher Domain: K/A/S/C Level Attained: K/KH/SH/P

Session: 10

Name(s) of the faculty: ______________________________

Date: ____________________ Time: ______________ to ______________

Duration: ____________________

Learning objective(s) of the session (Write from the presentation or as instructed by the faculty):

1. ______________________________
2. ______________________________
3. ______________________________
4. ______________________________

Teaching learning method(s) used in this session: ______________________________

Reflections

1. Please describe what happened during the session:

____

____

2. What did you learn in this session?

____

____

3. How do you think what you learnt in this session will be useful for you?

____

____

____

____

Signature of the Teacher Domain: K/A/S/C Level Attained: K/KH/SH/P

Session: 11

Name(s) of the faculty: ____________________

Date: ____________________ Time: ____________ to ____________

Duration: ____________________

Learning objective(s) of the session (Write from the presentation or as instructed by the faculty):

1. ____________________
2. ____________________
3. ____________________
4. ____________________

Teaching learning method(s) used in this session: ____________________

Reflections

1. Please describe what happened during the session:

____

____

2. What did you learn in this session?

____

____

3. How do you think what you learnt in this session will be useful for you?

____

____

____

____

Signature of the Teacher Domain: K/A/S/C Level Attained: K/KH/SH/P

Session: 12

Name(s) of the faculty: ______________________________

Date: ____________________   Time: ____________ to ____________

Duration: ____________________

Learning objective(s) of the session (Write from the presentation or as instructed by the faculty):

1. ______________________________
2. ______________________________
3. ______________________________
4. ______________________________

Teaching learning method(s) used in this session: ______________________________

Reflections

1. Please describe what happened during the session:

____

____

2. What did you learn in this session?

____

____

3. How do you think what you learnt in this session will be useful for you?

____

____

____

____

Signature of the Teacher   Domain: K/A/S/C   Level Attained: K/KH/SH/P

Session: 13

Name(s) of the faculty: ______________________________

Date: ____________________ Time: ____________ to ____________

Duration: ____________________

Learning objective(s) of the session (Write from the presentation or as instructed by the faculty):

1. ______________________________
2. ______________________________
3. ______________________________
4. ______________________________

Teaching learning method(s) used in this session: ______________________________

Reflections

1. Please describe what happened during the session:

____

____

2. What did you learn in this session?

____

____

3. How do you think what you learnt in this session will be useful for you?

____

____

____

____

Signature of the Teacher Domain: K/A/S/C Level Attained: K/KH/SH/P

Session: 14

Name(s) of the faculty: ____________________

Date: ____________________ Time: ____________ to ____________

Duration: ____________________

Learning objective(s) of the session (Write from the presentation or as instructed by the faculty):

1. ____________________
2. ____________________
3. ____________________
4. ____________________

Teaching learning method(s) used in this session: ____________________

Reflections

1. Please describe what happened during the session:

____

____

2. What did you learn in this session?

____

____

3. How do you think what you learnt in this session will be useful for you?

____

____

____

____

Signature of the Teacher Domain: K/A/S/C Level Attained: K/KH/SH/P

Session: 15

Name(s) of the faculty: ____________________

Date: ____________________ Time: ____________ to ____________

Duration: ____________________

Learning objective(s) of the session (Write from the presentation or as instructed by the faculty):

1. ____________________
2. ____________________
3. ____________________
4. ____________________

Teaching learning method(s) used in this session: ____________________

Reflections

1. Please describe what happened during the session:

____

____

2. What did you learn in this session?

____

____

3. How do you think what you learnt in this session will be useful for you?

____

____

____

____

Signature of the Teacher Domain: K/A/S/C Level Attained: K/KH/SH/P

Session: 16

Name(s) of the faculty: ________________________________

Date: ____________________ Time: ____________ to ____________

Duration: ____________________

Learning objective(s) of the session (Write from the presentation or as instructed by the faculty):

1. ________________________________
2. ________________________________
3. ________________________________
4. ________________________________

Teaching learning method(s) used in this session: ________________________________

Reflections

1. Please describe what happened during the session:

____

____

2. What did you learn in this session?

____

____

3. How do you think what you learnt in this session will be useful for you?

____

____

____

____

Signature of the Teacher Domain: K/A/S/C Level Attained: K/KH/SH/P

Session: 17

Name(s) of the faculty: ____________________

Date: ____________________ Time: ____________ to ____________

Duration: ____________________

Learning objective(s) of the session (Write from the presentation or as instructed by the faculty):

1. ____________________
2. ____________________
3. ____________________
4. ____________________

Teaching learning method(s) used in this session: ____________________

Reflections

1. Please describe what happened during the session:

____

____

2. What did you learn in this session?

____

____

3. How do you think what you learnt in this session will be useful for you?

____

____

____

____

Signature of the Teacher Domain: K/A/S/C Level Attained: K/KH/SH/P

Session: 18

Name(s) of the faculty: ____________________

Date: ____________________ Time: ____________ to ____________

Duration: ____________________

Learning objective(s) of the session (Write from the presentation or as instructed by the faculty):

1. ____________________
2. ____________________
3. ____________________
4. ____________________

Teaching learning method(s) used in this session: ____________________

Reflections

1. Please describe what happened during the session:

____

____

2. What did you learn in this session?

____

____

3. How do you think what you learnt in this session will be useful for you?

____

____

____

____

Signature of the Teacher Domain: K/A/S/C Level Attained: K/KH/SH/P

Session: 19

Name(s) of the faculty: ____________________

Date: ____________________ Time: ____________ to ____________

Duration: ____________________

Learning objective(s) of the session (Write from the presentation or as instructed by the faculty):

1. ____________________
2. ____________________
3. ____________________
4. ____________________

Teaching learning method(s) used in this session: ____________________

Reflections

1. Please describe what happened during the session:

____

____

2. What did you learn in this session?

____

____

3. How do you think what you learnt in this session will be useful for you?

____

____

____

____

Signature of the Teacher Domain: K/A/S/C Level Attained: K/KH/SH/P

Session: 20

Name(s) of the faculty: ______________________________

Date: ____________________ Time: ____________ to ____________

Duration: ____________________

Learning objective(s) of the session (Write from the presentation or as instructed by the faculty):

1. ______________________________
2. ______________________________
3. ______________________________
4. ______________________________

Teaching learning method(s) used in this session: ______________________________

Reflections

1. Please describe what happened during the session:

____

____

2. What did you learn in this session?

____

____

3. How do you think what you learnt in this session will be useful for you?

____

____

____

____

Signature of the Teacher Domain: K/A/S/C Level Attained: K/KH/SH/P

Session: 21

Name(s) of the faculty: ______________________________

Date: ____________________ Time: ____________ to ____________

Duration: ____________________

Learning objective(s) of the session (Write from the presentation or as instructed by the faculty):

1. ______________________________
2. ______________________________
3. ______________________________
4. ______________________________

Teaching learning method(s) used in this session: ______________________________

Reflections

1. Please describe what happened during the session:

____

____

2. What did you learn in this session?

____

____

3. How do you think what you learnt in this session will be useful for you?

____

____

____

____

Signature of the Teacher Domain: K/A/S/C Level Attained: K/KH/SH/P

Session: 22

Name(s) of the faculty: ______________________________

Date: ____________________ Time: ______________ to ______________

Duration: ____________________

Learning objective(s) of the session (Write from the presentation or as instructed by the faculty):

1. ______________________________
2. ______________________________
3. ______________________________
4. ______________________________

Teaching learning method(s) used in this session: ______________________________

Reflections

1. Please describe what happened during the session:

____

____

2. What did you learn in this session?

____

____

3. How do you think what you learnt in this session will be useful for you?

____

____

____

____

Signature of the Teacher Domain: K/A/S/C Level Attained: K/KH/SH/P

Session: 23

Name(s) of the faculty: ______________________________

Date: ____________________ Time: ____________ to ____________

Duration: ____________________

Learning objective(s) of the session (Write from the presentation or as instructed by the faculty):

1. ______________________________
2. ______________________________
3. ______________________________
4. ______________________________

Teaching learning method(s) used in this session: ______________________________

Reflections

1. Please describe what happened during the session:

____

____

2. What did you learn in this session?

____

____

3. How do you think what you learnt in this session will be useful for you?

____

____

____

____

Signature of the Teacher Domain: K/A/S/C Level Attained: K/KH/SH/P

Session: 24

Name(s) of the faculty: ____________________

Date: ____________________ Time: ____________ to ____________

Duration: ____________________

Learning objective(s) of the session (Write from the presentation or as instructed by the faculty):

1. ____________________
2. ____________________
3. ____________________
4. ____________________

Teaching learning method(s) used in this session: ____________________

Reflections

1. Please describe what happened during the session:

____

____

2. What did you learn in this session?

____

____

3. How do you think what you learnt in this session will be useful for you?

____

____

____

____

Signature of the Teacher Domain: K/A/S/C Level Attained: K/KH/SH/P

Session: 25

Name(s) of the faculty: ______________________________

Date: ______________ Time: ______________ to ______________

Duration: ______________

Learning objective(s) of the session (Write from the presentation or as instructed by the faculty):

1. ______________________________
2. ______________________________
3. ______________________________
4. ______________________________

Teaching learning method(s) used in this session: ______________________________

Reflections

1. Please describe what happened during the session:

____

____

2. What did you learn in this session?

____

____

3. How do you think what you learnt in this session will be useful for you?

____

____

____

____

Signature of the Teacher Domain: K/A/S/C Level Attained: K/KH/SH/P

Session: 26

Name(s) of the faculty: ____________________

Date: ____________________ Time: ____________ to ____________

Duration: ____________________

Learning objective(s) of the session (Write from the presentation or as instructed by the faculty):

1. ____________________
2. ____________________
3. ____________________
4. ____________________

Teaching learning method(s) used in this session: ____________________

Reflections

1. Please describe what happened during the session:

____

____

2. What did you learn in this session?

____

____

3. How do you think what you learnt in this session will be useful for you?

____

____

____

____

Signature of the Teacher Domain: K/A/S/C Level Attained: K/KH/SH/P

Session: 27

Name(s) of the faculty: ____________________

Date: ____________________ Time: ____________ to ____________

Duration: ____________________

Learning objective(s) of the session (Write from the presentation or as instructed by the faculty):

1. ____________________
2. ____________________
3. ____________________
4. ____________________

Teaching learning method(s) used in this session: ____________________

Reflections

1. Please describe what happened during the session:

____

____

2. What did you learn in this session?

____

____

3. How do you think what you learnt in this session will be useful for you?

____

____

____

____

Signature of the Teacher Domain: K/A/S/C Level Attained: K/KH/SH/P